Test of Integrated Language and Literacy Skills™ (TILLS™)

EXAMINER'S PRACTICE WORKBOOK

by

Nickola Wolf Nelson, Ph.D., CCC-SLP, BCS-CL
Western Michigan University
Kalamazoo

Elena Plante, Ph.D., CCC-SLP
The University of Arizona
Tucson

Nancy Helm-Estabrooks, Sc.D., CCC-SLP, BC-ANCDS
Western Carolina University
Cullowhee, North Carolina

and

Gillian Hotz, Ph.D., CCC-SLP
University of Miami
Miami, Florida

with contributions by

Michele A. Anderson, Ph.D., CCC-SLP
Western Michigan University
Kalamazoo

and

Michelle DeMaagd-Slager, M.A., CCC-SLP
Mary Free Bed Rehabilitation Hospital
Grand Rapids, Michigan

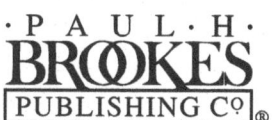

·P·A·U·L·H·
BROOKES
PUBLISHING Cº®

Baltimore • London • Sydney

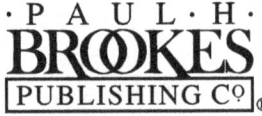

Paul H. Brookes Publishing Co.
Post Office Box 10624
Baltimore, Maryland 21285-0624

www.brookespublishing.com

Test of Integrated Language and Literacy Skills, TILLS, TILLS, and **TILLS Easy-Score**
are trademarks of Paul H. Brookes Publishing Co., Inc.

Typeset by Scribe Inc., Philadelphia, Pennsylvania.
Manufactured in the United States of America
by Potomac Printing Solutions, Inc., Landsdowne, Virginia.

The standardization research for the TILLS was supported by the Institute of Education Sciences,
U.S. Department of Education, through Grant R324A100354 to Western Michigan University. The
opinions expressed are those of the authors and do not represent views of the Institute or of the U.S.
Department of Education.

This workbook accompanies other components of the *Test of Integrated Language and Literacy Skills*™ (*TILLS*™).
For more information, contact Brookes Publishing Co., 1-800-638-3775; www.brookespublishing.com/tills.

Library of Congress Control Number: 2015948336
ISBN-13: 978-1-59857-913-0
ISBN-10: 1-59857-913-4

2024   2023

10   9

Contents

Overview

The *Test of Integrated Language and Literacy Skills™ (TILLS™) Examiner's Practice Workbook* provides instructions and scoring practice for the TILLS. It is designed to be used in conjunction with the *TILLS Examiner's Manual*. We recommend that you read Chapter 2 of the *Examiner's Manual* first and keep that manual open while completing the exercises in this *Examiner's Practice Workbook*. The *TILLS Quick Start Guide* also summarizes the key information related to administering each subtest. By working through the practice exercises in this workbook, you will reinforce your understanding of how to use the standardized procedures to administer and score the 15 TILLS subtests.

The outline of subtests within the TILLS test model appears in Table 1. Practice exercises for each of these subtests constitute Section I of this workbook. Sections IIA and IIB provide practice in transforming raw scores to standard scores and practice in interpreting TILLS results for its three validated purposes. While working on these two sections, you will need to refer to Chapter 3 in the *Examiner's Manual*.

Some of the practice exercises involve listening to and scoring samples of students' spoken responses. You will find these in the *TILLS Digital Audio Files* (on the USB drive that comes with your *TILLS Examiner's Kit*) in the folder labeled Examiner's Practice Workbook Audio Files on Tracks 1–14. TILLS subtests with oral language responses are

- Track 1 Vocabulary Awareness (VA) Practice Example

- Track 2 Phonemic Awareness (PA) Practice Example

- Track 3 Story Retelling (SRa) Story A Practice Exercise

- Track 4 Story Retelling (SRb) Story B Practice Exercise

Table 1. The TILLS language levels-by-modalities model (plus memory) and related subtests

Language modality	Language level	
	Sound/word level	Sentence/discourse level
Listening	1. Vocabulary Awareness (VA)* 2. Phonemic Awareness (PA)	6. Listening Comprehension (LC) 8. Following Directions (FD)
Speaking	4. Nonword Repetition (NWRep)	3. Story Retelling (SR) 13. Social Communication (SC)
Reading	10. Nonword Reading (NWRead) 11. Reading Fluency (RF)	7. Reading Comprehension (RC)
Writing	5. Nonword Spelling (NWSpell) 12a. Written Expression–Word Score (WE-Word)	12b. Written Expression–Discourse Score (WE-Disc) 12c. Written Expression–Sentence Score (WE-Sent)
Memory	14. Digit Span Forward (DSF) 15. Digit Span Backward (DSB)	9. Delayed Story Retelling (DSR)

*The Vocabulary Awareness (VA) subtest uses word-level stimuli; this subtest, however, assesses semantic relations. As such, it is statistically related to sentence/discourse skills. See Chapter 2 of the *TILLS Technical Manual* for more information.

- Track 5 Nonword Repetition (NWRep) Practice Exercise

- Track 6 Listening Comprehension (LC) Practice Exercise

- Track 7 Reading Comprehension (RC) Practice Exercise

- Track 8 Delayed Story Retelling (DSRa) Story A Practice Exercise

- Track 9 Delayed Story Retelling (DSRb) Story B Practice Exercise

- Track 10 Nonword Reading (NWRead) Practice Exercise

- Track 11 Reading Fluency (RF) Practice Exercise

- Track 12 Social Communication (SC) Practice Exercise

- Track 13 Digit Span Forward (DSF) Practice Exercise

- Track 14 Digit Span Backward (DSB) Practice Exercise

Practice samples for subtests that require written responses are provided in this workbook. TILLS subtests that require written responses are

- Nonword Spelling (NWSpell)

- Following Directions (FD)

- Reading Comprehension (RC)

- Written Expression (WE)

Scoring the Written Expression (WE) subtest requires a grammatical skill that may be new to some examiners. That is, to calculate the Written Expression–Sentence score (WE-Sent), examiners must first divide students' written language samples into T-units (independent clauses with embedded or subordinate clauses and phrases). Section III includes a tutorial on syntactic structure and T-unit division. If this is an unfamiliar skill, you should complete this tutorial before you complete the practice exercises. Section III also includes additional scored examples from the WE subtest.

You will need a blank *TILLS Examiner Record Form* to record your answers to the practice exercises and then compare your answers to the filled-in *Examiner Record Form* examples. For each exercise, do not read the Answers section until you have completed the exercise.

After you complete all the practice exercises, you can keep this workbook as a resource to refer to as you administer the TILLS over time. It serves as a helpful reminder of administration rules and can help you check your fidelity.

SECTION I

SECTION I

Practice Exercises for the 15 TILLS Subtests

This section provides exercises for each of the 15 subtests of the *Test of Integrated Language and Literacy Skills™ (TILLS™)*, along with a brief summary of each subtest's instructions.

SUBTEST 1: Vocabulary Awareness (VA)

RECAP OF SUBTEST

In the Vocabulary Awareness (VA) subtest, the student is shown a set of three printed words in the *TILLS Stimulus Book* while the examiner reads them aloud. Then, the student is asked to pick two of the words that go together and explain why. Next, the student is asked to choose a different pair of words from the same set that go together in a different way and explain why they go together.

Use as a stand-alone measure: Yes

Average time to administer: 15 minutes

Materials: *Examiner Record Form* (pp. 2–4), *Stimulus Book* (pp. 3–55)

Start rule: Start points for age ranges are indicated by arrows.

Basal rule: 4 consecutive scores of 2 (both parts of each item must be correct)

Ceiling rule: 6 scores of 0 within a sequence of 8 consecutive items (both parts of each item must be incorrect on 6 out of 8 items)

Repetition: Allowed

Probes: Yes (as specified in the *Examiner's Manual*)

PRACTICE EXERCISE

To complete this exercise, you will need Track 1 from the Examiner's Practice Workbook Audio Files folder on the *TILLS Digital Audio Files* (USB drive) for Student 1, a 6-year, 9-month-old boy with normal language. Listen to the test administration on the audio file and score Student 1's responses using a blank *Examiner Record Form*.

Ask yourself the following questions as you complete the exercise:

1. What must I do to establish a basal for this student?

2. What must I do to establish a ceiling for this student? What should I do if I mistakenly tested beyond the ceiling and the student answered an item above the ceiling correctly? Does it score as a 1 or a 0?

3. What should I do if the student said two words "mean the same"?

4. Which items are the most challenging to score? What rationale guides my decisions?

ANSWERS

Make your best effort to complete the exercise before you read the following answers:

1. Nothing is required to establish a basal for Student 1 because testing with this 6-year, 9-month-old boy begins with Item 1. Therefore, 1 is the basal.

2. The ceiling rule applies. As the sample *Examiner Record Form* shows, the examiner ceases testing after Item 23, but she could end on Item 22 because Student 1 has earned 0 on both parts of 6 out of 8 consecutive items at that point (Items 15, 18, 19, 20, 21, and 22). Note that this ceiling rule requires that the student miss both parts of the two-part VA items to count as 0. If any student gets an item correct past the ceiling, you must count it as 0. In this example, you would have had to score Item 23 as 0, even if Student 1 had gotten it right because it was past the ceiling.

3. You should use the probe "Can you tell me what they mean?" when Student 1 says two words "mean the same." An example of this occurs on Item 5a, when he says that *bark* and *growl* mean the same thing.

4. Challenging items include the following, with notes about rationale for decisions made.

   • *Item 3b:* Score 1 for *airplane* and *train* because "both electrical" captures the idea of being powered, which does not apply to kite.

   • *Item 5a:* Score 1 for *bark* and *growl* because the response to the probe after the initial answer "mean the same" was "bark means a dog is mad; growl means a dog is mad." This expresses the intended meaning that both are sounds a dog makes.

   • *Item 5b:* Score 0 for *bark* and *tree* because "dogs sometimes like to bark at trees" misses the part–whole meaning of bark being part of a tree.

   • *Item 15b:* Score 0 for *knee* and *elbow* because "you can both use your knee and elbow in soccer" misses the categorical meaning that they are both joints; that reason also applies to foot.

   • *Item 17b:* Score 0 for *step* and *stair* because "you can step down or up on stairs" does not recognize that *step* is a part of *stairs,* or *steps* is another name for *stairs.* Note also that you can also *march* up or down stairs.

Practice Items

dog–cat–**bone**	dog–cat–**bone**
Both animals / pets *dogs chase cats* coach	Dogs like / eat / chew / bury bones
light–sun–feather	**light–sun**–**feather**
Sun gives light / both bright	Feather is light / not heavy *coached double meaning*

Subtest Items   Total Item Score (a + b)

1a.	**pen–pig–paper**	0	(1)	1b.	**pen–pig**–paper	(0)	1	1
6–11	Use pen to write on paper				Keep a pig in a pen *DK [don't know]*			

2a.	**thorn–rose**–daisy	0	(1)	2b.	thorn–**rose–daisy**	0	(1)	2
	Roses have thorns *thorns grow on roses*				Both flowers			

3a.	**kite–airplane**–train	0	(1)	3b.	kite–**airplane–train**	0	(1)	2
	Both fly / go in sky (*not* a kite can be shaped like an airplane)				Both transportation / carry people / can ride in them Both have wheels / engines / use electricity / are machines (*not* you can take airplanes on a train)			

4a.	**saw–hammer**–eyes	0	(1)	4b.	saw–hammer–**eyes**	(0)	1	1
	Both tools / have handles				Eyes for seeing / I saw with my eyes *DK*			

5a.	**bark–growl**–tree	0	(1)	5b.	**bark–growl–tree**	(0)	1	1
12–13	Both sounds a dog makes *"Mean same thing"* *bark/growl means a dog is mad*				Bark covers / grows on tree *"dogs sometimes like to bark at trees" (not central meaning)*			

6a.	**taste**–nose–**smell**	(0)	1	6b.	taste–**nose–smell**	0	(1)	1
	Both senses (*not* you can smell and taste food) *can taste better when you can smell*				Smell with nose / use nose to smell			

7a.	**oven**–ice cream–**freezer**	(0)	1	7b.	oven–**ice cream–freezer**	0	(1)	1
14+	Both appliances / make food hot or cold (*not* in the kitchen)				Ice cream goes in freezer *both really cold*			

8a.	**painter**–elevator–**ladder**	0	(1)	8b.	painter–**elevator–ladder**	0	(1)	2
	Painter uses / stands on ladder / paints with a ladder / needs a ladder to paint. *General prompt not to quit too soon*				Use to go up / reach high places *both take you up*			

9a.	**stomach–swallow**–cardinal	0	(1)	9b.	stomach–**swallow–cardinal**	(0)	1	1
	When swallowed, food goes to stomach				Both birds *DK*			

10a.	**sphinx–pyramid**–triangle	(0)	1	10b.	sphinx–**pyramid–triangle**	0	(1)	1
	Both found in Egypt / in desert *DK* Both ancient				Pyramid is shaped like triangle Both shapes			

11a.	**left**–correct–**right**	0	(1)	11b.	left–**correct–right**	(0)	1	1
	Tell opposite directions (or gestures to show) *both sides*				Both describe picking a good answer / *DK* making a good choice			

12a.	**diamond–baseball**–ruby	(0)	1	12b.	diamond–**baseball–ruby**	0	(1)	1
	Play baseball on a diamond / baseball field called *DK* diamond				Both jewels / rocks / gems / minerals *both shine* Both shiny / expensive / come from mines *[major shared characteristic]*			

13a.	**bat–owl**–eagle	0	(1)	13b.	bat–**owl–eagle**	(0)	1	1
	Nocturnal, up at night (*not* predators)				Both birds / have feathers / have beaks / have talons / make nests (*not* predators) *used probe because student said "all both fly" when*			

reminded to pick two that go together in way third does not

5

14a.	hammer–hatchet–tree	0	(1)		14b.	hammer–hatchet–tree	(0)	1	I
Both tools / have handles					Use hatchet to cut down tree *DK what hatchet is*				

15a.	knee–foot–elbow	(0)	1		15b.	knee–foot–elbow	(0)	1	O
Both on leg / used to walk					Both bend / are joints (*not* have round knobs or are hard) *can both use your knee and elbow in soccer*				

16a.	fan–propeller–admirer	0	(1)		16b.	fan–propeller–admirer	(0)	1	I
Both have blades / go around / move air A fan has a propeller (can gesture spinning) *both spin around*					Both mean to like something / someone *DK*				

17a.	march–step–stair	0	(1)		17b.	march–step–stair	(0)	1	I
Marching is a / uses a special kind of step / stepping in rhythm *"You step to march"*					Both parts of a staircase / for going up or down a level in a building / step is part of a stair *"Step down or up on stairs"* (*not* you can step upstairs; must get noun meaning) *(doesn't count because could also march up stairs)*				

18a.	scales–ounce–thermometer	(0)	1		18b.	scales–ounce–thermometer	(0)	1	O
Both are related to weight / weigh ounces with a scale *DK*					Both used to measure / thermometer has a scale / in a doctor's office *DK*				

19a.	canary–banana–hawk	(0)	1		19b.	canary–banana–hawk	(0)	1	O
Both yellow / found in tropics (*not* canaries eat bananas) *DK*					Both birds				

20a.	capsule–pill–spaceship	(0)	1		20b.	capsule–pill–spaceship	(0)	1	O
Both used for space travel / capsule is part of spaceship / astronaut rides in the capsule					Both medicine you swallow / pill can take form of capsule / pills are in capsules *DK*				

21a.	trout–flounder–struggle	(0)	1		21b.	trout–flounder–struggle	(0)	1	O
Both fish *struggle to catch a trout.*					Both mean having trouble / difficulty with something				

22a.	plum–cut–prune	(0)	1		22b.	plum–cut–prune	(0)	1	O
Both fruit / prune is a dried plum *DK*					Both mean to use something sharp to slice / cut (*not* you can cut a prune or plum) *Ceiling*				

23a.	conceal–hide–skin	(0)	1		23b.	conceal–hide–skin	(0)	1	O
Both mean to keep out of sight Conceal means you're going to hide something (*not* your skin conceals your bones) *DK*					Both cover body / animals (*not* you use concealer on your skin)				

24a.	mean–average–spite	0	1		24b.	mean–average–spite	0	1	
Both terms for computing a number / telling the middle number / used in math					Both describe person who is not nice / tries to get back at someone				

25a.	nylon–plastic–cotton	0	1		25b.	nylon–plastic–cotton	0	1	
Both synthetic / manmade / made from petroleum					Both types of fabric / used for clothing				

Total score: __19__ / 50

Qualitative observations:

Vocabulary Awareness (VA) subtest scored for Student 1, a 6-year, 9-month-old boy.

SUBTEST 2: Phonemic Awareness (PA)

RECAP OF SUBTEST

In the Phonemic Awareness (PA) subtest, the student is asked to listen to a nonword and repeat it without the initial phoneme.

Use as a stand-alone measure: Yes
Average time to administer: 3 minutes
Materials: *Examiner Record Form* (pp. 5–6), audio recording device (recommended)
Start rule: Start points for age ranges are indicated by arrows.

Basal rule: 6 consecutive scores of 1
Ceiling rule: Scores 0 on 6 out of 8 consecutive items
Repetition: No (unless ambient noise interferes)
Probes: None

PRACTICE EXERCISE

To complete this exercise, you will need Track 2 from the Examiner's Practice Workbook Audio Files folder on the *Digital Audio Files* (USB drive) for Student 1, a 6-year, 9-month-old boy with normal language. Listen to the test administration on the audio file and score Student 1's responses using a blank *Examiner Record Form*. Note that it is acceptable to record differences in the student's response from the target correct response using standard orthography, using International Phonetic Alphabet (IPA) symbols, or marking changes on either spelling in the *Examiner Record Form*. It is important to have good phonemic awareness skills to administer and score this test, but it is not necessary to know the IPA. You can find descriptions of the IPA on the Internet.

In addition, you might find it helpful to listen to Track 1 in the Phonemic Awareness (PA) Audio files demo folder in the *Digital Audio Files*.

Ask yourself the following questions as you complete the exercise:

1. What must I do to establish a basal for this student?

2. What must I do to establish a ceiling for this student?

3. What error does the examiner make in administering Item 3?

4. What rule does the examiner follow correctly in administering Items 12 and 19?

5. Which items are the most challenging to score? What rationale do I need to guide my decisions?

6. Student 1 responds correctly to Item 22. Students who are using a spelling strategy to respond to this item tend to answer it incorrectly. What response would you expect a student to make to Item 22 if he or she were using a spelling strategy?

ANSWERS

Make your best effort to complete the exercise before you read the following answers:

1. Nothing is required to establish a basal for this student because testing a 6-year, 9-month-old begins with Item 1. Therefore, 1 is the basal.

2. The ceiling rule applies. Student 1 comes close to establishing a ceiling when he misses five in a row (Items 9–13); however, he gets the next five items correct, and he never reaches a ceiling of 0 on 6 out of 8 consecutive items, so all 22 items are administered.

3. The examiner makes an error while administering Item 3 when she misses hearing the student's original production and has to ask for a repetition. In this case, listening to the recording revealed that the student did not alter his response. If he had, the examiner should score the first response from the audio recording rather than the requested repetition. If a student makes a spontaneous self-correction (marked "sc"), score the student's self-corrected response. In general, score the student's final response, whether it is correct or incorrect.

4. On Item 12, Student 1 makes a noise with his chair that interferes with his ability to hear the test item, "glem," so the examiner repeats it; however, there is no noise coincidental with Item 19, "strid," so when he asks for a repetition on that item, the examiner says, "Sorry, I can't repeat that one."

5. Challenging items included the following, with notes about rationale for decisions made.

   • *Item 1:* Score 0 for Item 1 because Student 1 adds an /l/.

   • *Item 11:* Score 0 for "brogger" becomes "rogger" because the student includes a consonant (sounded like /b/) at the beginning of the revised word.

   • *Item 13:* Score 0 for Item 13. Student 1 correctly removes /h/ from the initial position in the word, but he also removes the /t/ from the end of the word. Any change in the word other than initial consonant deletion is counted as an error. The only exceptions to this rule are if the change represents an articulatory pattern or dialectal shift in pronunciation that appears consistently in the student's spontaneous speech.

   • *Item 20:* Score 0 for Item 20. Although Student 1 correctly removes /s/ from the initial position in the word, he inserts a phoneme (sounded like /f/ or /p/) in the portion of the word that remains. A tip for the examiner is to watch the student's lips when assessing responses.

6. Student 1 responds correctly to Item 22 by saying "apet," showing removal of the initial phoneme /tʃ/. This single phoneme is represented by two letters, "ch." Therefore, students who are using a spelling strategy rather than a phoneme strategy to respond to this item are likely to leave the /h/ at the beginning of the revised word (removing only one letter rather than one sound). Such a student would say "hapet," which is an incorrect response and scores 0.

Subtest Items

Item	Phonetic spelling	Spoken response	Score	
6–7 1. dop → op	/dɑp / → /ɑp /	lap	(0)	1
2. bap → ap	/bæp / → /æp /		0	(1)
3. blom → lom	/blɑm/ → /lɑm/	am	(0)	1
4. molk → olk	/molk/ → /olk/		0	(1)
5. gilf → ilf	/gɪlf/ → /ɪlf/		0	(1)
6. flig → lig	/flɪg / → /lɪg /		0	(1)
7. lekel → ekel	/lɛkəl/ → /ɛkəl/		0	(1)
8–14 8. krit → rit	/krɪt/ → /rɪt/		0	(1)
9. swog → wog	/swɔg / → /wɔg /	ɔg	(0)	1
10. treeg → reeg	/trig/ → /rig/	ig	(0)	1
15+ 11. brogger → rogger	/brɑgɚ/ → /rɑgɚ/	brɑgɚ	(0)	1
12. glem → lem	/glɛm/ → /lɛm/	ɪm	(0)	1
13. hidot → idot	/hāɪdɑt/ → /āɪdɑt/	aɪdʌ	(0)	1
14. wookup → ookup	/wukʌp/ → /ukʌp/		0	(1)

Note that it is not optimal to ask for repetition by the child. Fortunately child did not revise response in this case.

Examiner repeated this word due to interference of ambient noise.

Error on final sound counts. Must repeat remainder of word accurately.

(FORM PAGE BREAK)

Item	Phonetic spelling	Spoken response	Score	
15. cramset → ramset	/kræmsɛt/ → /ræmsɛt/		0	(1)
16. frab → rab	/fræb/ → /ræb/		0	(1)
17. slooslom → looslom	/sluslɑm/ → /luslɑm/		0	(1)
18. repuze → epuze	/ripjuz/ → /ipjuz/		0	(1)
19. strid → trid	/strɪd/ → /trɪd/	/t/	(0)	1
20. strat → trat	/stræt/ → /træt/	/træpt/	(0)	1
21. striggler → triggler	/strɪglɚ/ → /trɪglɚ/		0	(1)
22. chapet → apet	/ʧæpət/ → /æpət/		0	(1)

Note: Child asked for repetition. Examiner said, "I can't repeat that one" (Not due to ambient noise)

Total score: 13 / 22

Qualitative observations:

Phonemic Awareness (PA) subtest scored for Student 1, a 6-year, 9-month-old boy.

SUBTEST 3: Story Retelling (SR)

RECAP OF SUBTEST

In the Story Retelling (SR) subtest, the student is asked to listen to an age-appropriate story and retell it.

Use as a stand-along measure: Yes (*Note:* Subtest 3 can be used as a stand-alone measure or in conjunction with Subtest 9. If administered together with Subtest 9, Subtest 3 must be administered approximately 20-30 minutes before Subtest 9, with language-related activities intervening.)

Average time to administer: 4 minutes

Materials: *Examiner Record Form* (pp. 7–10), audio recording device (recommended)

Story A: "Tommy the Trickster" for ages 6;0–11;11 (p. 7 of the *Examiner Record Form*)

Story B: "The Rubber Raft" for ages 12;0–18;11 (p. 9 of the *Examiner Record Form*)

Start rule: Arrows with age ranges in years indicate which story to administer

Basal rule: None

Ceiling rule: None

Repetition: No (unless ambient noise interferes)

Probes: Yes (as specified in the *Examiner's Manual*)

PRACTICE EXERCISE

To complete this exercise, you will need Track 3 from the Examiner's Practice Workbook Audio Files folder on the *Digital Audio Files* (USB drive) for Student 1, a 6-year, 9-month-old boy with normal language, and Track 4 for Student 2, a 13-year-old boy with moderate-severe bilateral sensorineural hearing loss who uses binaural digital hearing aids. Listen to the audio files for the two students retelling Story A and Story B. Using a blank *Examiner Record Form,* score the 6-year, 9-month-old student's responses for Story A. Score the 13-year-old student's responses for Story B. You may want to listen to each story more than once to confirm your scoring. Be sure to score the answers to the comprehension questions as well as scoring the stories themselves. When scoring the student's retelling, just circle 1 as you listen to the story. Do not circle 0 for any missing content units until later (or skip this step altogether). The reasons for this are two-fold. First, it saves time. Second, some students (Student 2, for example) revise their story as they go. When a student later adds a content unit you thought that he or she had missed, you can circle 1 without having to cross out 0 for that item.

Ask yourself the following questions as you complete the exercise:

1. What basal and ceiling rules apply when administering Stories A and B?

2. What general prompt is allowed when administering these stories, which the examiner used when administering Story A?

3. Are there any probes for specific information that are acceptable when administering these stories?

4. What synonyms do the two students use in retelling the two stories that I should credit? When do I need to apply the general rule, "When in doubt, give credit"?

5. What self-talk do I hear the 13-year-old use when answering Comprehension Question 2, which shows good prognosis even though he could not answer the question correctly?

6. According to the *Examiner's Manual,* at what age do students typically answer all four questions correctly?

ANSWERS

Make your best effort to complete the exercise before you read the following answers:

1. The SR subtest has no basal or ceiling for either age group.

2. The examiner uses the general prompt "Is there more?" to ask the student retelling Story A whether he is done.

3. No other specific probes are allowed.

4. The two students use several acceptable synonyms:

   - *Story A, Items 4–7:* Student 1 earns credit for Items 4–7 by describing how he got fat because he ate so much junk food, even though he modifies the wording and verb tense slightly because he maintains the original meaning and incorporates the content of these items.

   - *Story A, Item 9:* "Stuffed" earns credit as a synonym of "stocked."

   - *Story A, Items 12 and 26:* "Vegetables" counts as a superordinate for "carrot sticks."

   - *Story A, Item 19:* "He said" counts for "he told."

   - *Story A, Item 22:* "are not good" counts for "were bad."

   - *Story B, Items 16–20:* Scoring for Student 2 is a bit tricky because he retells several elements out of order. He earns credit for these items because reordering does not influence correctness as long as the essence of the original meaning is maintained.

   - *Story B, Item 18:* Student 2 uses words from the original story, "By the time," to earn credit for Item 18, but he also would have earned credit if he had said "After" to describe completion of pumping up the raft.

   - *Story B, Item 33:* Student 2 earns credit for "they were walking back" by saying, "when they got back." One could argue that this shifts the meaning slightly, but it captures the essence and follows the general rule to give credit when in doubt.

   - *Story B, Item 50:* The examiner decided to give credit for "plastic" in place of rubber because manufactured rubber and plastic are related and blow-up rafts may be made of plastic. This follows the general rule to give credit when in doubt; however, a note might be made under Qualitative Observations to look more closely at the student's vocabulary and word-retrieval skills.

5. When answering Comprehension Question 2, the 13-year-old says quietly to himself, "That's the one I had a problem with." This shows that he is aware he missed a piece of the story, and further, that it is the piece he needs to answer the question about what the activity leader had told Michael and Angie they had to do. This is an indicator of Student 2's ability to use executive functions to monitor his comprehension.

6. The information in the *Examiner's Manual* indicates that students with normal language should be able to answer all four questions correctly by age 9. Missing one question, by itself, does not signal disorder, but the criterion reference is to get all four questions correct by age 9 years. If students who are 9 years old or older cannot answer one or more of the comprehension questions, other indicators of possible comprehension difficulties should be examined using data from other TILLS subtests, teacher and parent reports (e.g., *TILLS Student Language Scale [SLS]*), and curriculum-based language assessment.

Content Units	Score	
1. Tommy's (must use proper name to count on first instance)	0	(1)
2. mother	(0)	1
3. thought he (Tommy, worried)	(0)	1
4. was getting fat (bigger, gaining weight) got fat	0	(1)
5. from eating he ate	0	(1)
6. too much so much	0	(1)
7. junk food (cookies)	0	(1)
8. so she Mom	0	(1)
9. stocked (put) stuffed	0	(1)
10. the refrigerator (fridge, icebox)	0	(1)
11. fruit (healthy foods [only scores once] [not grapes, etc.*])	0	(1)
12. carrots (carrot sticks, healthy foods, vegetables)	0	(1)
13. she even put	(0)	1
14. these things	(0)	1
15. in his lunchbox (lunch bag, lunch)	(0)	1
16. but Tommy (he)	(0)	1
17. was a "fast talker" (figurative meaning)	(0)	1

Content Units	Score	
18. at school	0	(1)
19. he convinced (talked them into, told) said	0	(1)
20. his friends	0	(1)
21. that cookies	0	(1)
22. were bad are not good	0	(1)
23. for them	0	(1)
24. then he traded	0	(1)
25. his fruit (healthy foods [only scores once])	0	(1)
26. carrots (carrot sticks, healthy foods) vegetables	0	(1)
27. for cookies → prompt for more	0	(1)
28. his mother	0	(1)
29. didn't know why	0	(1)
30. Tommy (he)	0	(1)
31. kept gaining weight (getting bigger/fatter)	0	(1)
32. when all she had given him	(0)	1
33. were healthy foods	(0)	1

*The scoring guideline is that a child can get credit for a superordinate category label (*vegetables* for *carrots*) but not a more specific one (e.g., *grapes* for *fruit* does not earn credit).

Total score: __24__ / 33

Comprehension Questions

Question	Score	
1. Why did Tommy's mother worry about him?		
She thought he was getting fat/gaining weight. Because he kept getting fat	0	(1)
2. How did Tommy trick his mother?		
By trading his healthy foods for his friends' cookies. At school he traded his fruits and vegetables for their junk food and cookies.	0	(1)
3. Why did Tommy's mother feel confused?		
Because she was giving him healthy foods but he was still gaining weight. Because he didn't know that he was trading his fruits and vegetables for the cookies	0	(1)
4. In the story you heard that Tommy was a fast talker. What do you think that meant?		
He was good at talking people into things/convincing/persuasive (*not* he could talk very fast). That ... he ... I don't know how to explain it.	(0)	1

Note: Credit variations that maintain the intended meaning

Comprehension questions score: __3__ / 4

Qualitative observations:

fruits pronounced /frutst/

Story Retelling (SR) subtest (Story A) scored for Student 1, a 6-year, 9-month-old boy.

Content Units	Score	
1. (last) summer	(0)	1
2. Michael (must use proper name)	0	(1)
3. Angie (must use proper name)	0	(1)
4. went	0	(1)
5. to the lake (beach)	0	(1)
6. at the park	0	(1)
7. when they got there	(0)	1
8. they asked	0	(1)
9. activity	0	(1)
10. leader (accept synonyms [only scores once]) director	0	(1)
11. if they could use	0	(1)
12. one	(0)	1
13. of the rubber rafts lake raft	0	(1)
14. he said	(0)	1
15. they could (yes)	0	1
16. if they would	0	1
17. pump it up (blow it up, inflate it)	0	1
18. by the time	0	(1)
19. they finished	(0)	1
20. inflating (pumping up, blowing it up) they pump up	0	(1)
21. the raft (rubber boat, rubber thing)	0	(1)
22. Michael (the kids/they [only scores once])	0	(1)
23. Angie (the kids)	(0)	1
24. were tired	0	(1)
25. and thirsty	0	(1)
26. so they left	(0)	1

Content Units	Score	
27. the raft	(0)	1
28. by the lake	(0)	1
29. while they went	0	(1)
30. to the snack bar	(0)	1
31. for a drink got something to drink	0	(1)
32. as (while/when) by the time	0	(1)
33. they were walking back they got back	0	(1)
34. they spotted (saw)	(0)	1
35. a huge (large)	(0)	1
36. gray There was a gray	0	(1)
37. cat cat.	0	(1)
38. with claws out	(0)	1
39. getting ready	0	(1)
40. to pounce	0	(1)
41. on the raft	0	(1)
42. they started running	0	(1)
43. toward the raft	0	(1)
44. yelling at	(0)	1
45. the cat	(0)	1
46. (but) by the time (when)	0	(1)
47. they got there	0	(1)
48. it was too late	(0)	1
49. they were looking at	0	(1)
50. a rubber plastic	0	(1)
51. pancake	0	(1)

Total score: 32 / 51

Comprehension Questions

Question	Score	
1. What did Michael and Angie ask the activity leader?		
If they could borrow a raft If they can use the lake raft.	0	(1)
2. What did the activity leader tell them they had to do?		
Pump it up/inflate the raft (That's the one I had problem with) They had to take care of it	(0)	1
3. Why were they tired and thirsty?		
Because they worked hard to blow up the raft Because they had to pump all the air into the raft.	0	(1)
4. In the story you heard that Michael and Angie saw a rubber pancake. What do you think that meant?		
The raft was flat/looked like a pancake/the cat popped the raft The raft was deflated by the cat, well pretty much the cat … (trailed off)	0	(1)

Comprehension questions score: 3 /4

Qualitative observations:

Story Retelling (SR) subtest (Story B) scored for Student 2, a 13-year-old boy.

SUBTEST 4: Nonword Repetition (NWRep)

RECAP OF SUBTEST

In the Nonword Repetition (NWRep) subtest, the student is asked to listen to non-words delivered via digital recording and repeat them.

Use as a stand-along measure: Yes (**Note:** Subtest 4 can be used as a stand-alone measure or in conjunction with Subtest 5. If administered together with Subtest 5, Subtest 4 must be administered immediately before Subtest 5 and in the same session.)

Average time to administer: 4 minutes

Materials: *Examiner Record Form* (pp. 11–12), audio player, *Digital Audio Files* (Tracks 2–28), audio recording device (recommended)

Start rule: Start at the beginning for all students.

Basal rule: None

Ceiling rule: Scores 0 on 6 out of 8 consecutive items

Repetition: No (unless ambient noise interferes)

Probes: None

PRACTICE EXERCISE

To complete this exercise, you will need Track 5 from the Examiner's Practice Work-book Audio Files folder on the *Digital Audio Files* (USB drive) for Student 1, a 6-year, 9-month-old boy with normal language. Listen to the test administration on the audio file and score Student 1's responses using a blank *Examiner Record Form*. Note that target spoken responses for this subtest are presented using International Phonetic Alphabet (IPA) symbols; however, it is acceptable to record differences in a student's response from the target correct response using standard orthography (i.e., letters) or by marking changes, such as substituted, inserted, or deleted phonemes, on either the orthographic spelling or phonetic representation in the *Examiner Record Form*. It is important to have good phonemic awareness skills to administer and score this test, but it is not necessary to know the IPA. You can find descriptions of the IPA on the Internet.

Ask yourself the following questions as you complete the exercise:

1. What must I do to establish a basal for this 6-year, 9-month-old student? How would this differ if the student were 12 years old?

2. What must I do to establish a ceiling for this 6-year, 9-month-old student?

3. What special steps should I take when administering the NWRep and Nonword Spelling (NWSpell) subtests to students with hearing loss?

4. Are there any conditions under which I would give credit (score 1) to a student's imitative response, even if it involves a change in word pronunciation, such as a modification of a vowel or voicing (or devoicing) of consonants?

5. What items does Student 1 repeat incorrectly, and what changes does he make that made them incorrect?

ANSWERS

Make your best effort to complete the exercise before you read the following answers:

1. For the NWRep subtest, all students start at the beginning of the recording, regardless of age, because of the difficulty of testing backward when using the digital recording. Therefore, you should start the audio stimuli on Track 2, Intro-duction, on the *Digital Audio Files*. Next, present the two practice items; then, continue with Item 1 for all students. This rule would not differ for a student age 12 or older. You usually will not need to pause the audio recording when present-ing test items on this subtest.

2. You can stop testing if a student has earned 0 on 6 out of 8 consecutive items. This is the ceiling rule for all students; however, you may want to continue testing to gain additional qualitative information about a given student's speech perception and repetition skills, particularly when assessing a student who is deaf or hard of hearing or any student who makes extensive errors on this subtest. Most school-age students with normal language who take the TILLS can complete the NWRep task with few errors. If you continue testing beyond the ceiling, you must score all items above the ceiling as 0. This allows you to compare the student's raw score on the subtest with normative data and to transform raw scores to standard scores.

3. For all students, testing should be completed in a room that is free from the adverse effects of background noise and reverberation on speech understanding. A digital audio player with high-quality speakers and volume control should be used. Adjust the volume so that it is comfortably loud for the student. For students who are deaf or hard of hearing, examiners should ensure that students are wearing their hearing technology and that it is in good working order. External speakers or remote microphone technology such as an FM system or Bluetooth microphone device may be utilized.

4. Any changes in word pronunciation involving vowels; consonant voicing (or devoicing); or phoneme substitutions, additions, deletions, or transposition count as errors unless they can be attributed to consistent misarticulations or dialect differences. Consistent with this rule, you should assign a score of 1 to any item if the student makes a change that is consistent with his or her spontaneous speech pattern. For example, regional or ethnic differences may affect pronunciations of vowels, making them more tense (e.g., /ɛ/ goes to /i/) or more lax (e.g., /o/ goes to /ə/) or turning vowels into diphthongs (e.g., /i/ goes to /iə/). Speakers of African American English may devoice final voiced consonants so that /d/ on "gid" sounds close to a /t/, but without the aspirated puff of air at the end, or the /b/ on "dabe" sounds close to a /p/. Speakers of Spanish-influenced English may reduce the affrication on "ch," pronouncing "smitchly" to sound more like "smishly." Speakers of Asian-influenced English could have difficulty with the /r/ and /l/ phonemes. Count any such changes as errors unless you have evidence that they are produced in that manner consistently in the student's spontaneous speech. Student 1 makes few errors, and none of them can be attributed to articulatory difficulties or dialectal differences.

5. The errors can be listed and analyzed as follows:

   • *Item 10:* Student 1 devoices the /g/ in "untigament," saying "untikament" instead, scoring 0 on this item.

   • *Item 11:* Student 1 changes the vowel from /skroil/ to /skrɛl/, scoring 0 on this item.

   • *Item 15:* Student 1 reproduces this item correctly, scoring 1, but it is not unusual for students to voice the "ch" to sound like "dg," pronouncing "smitchly" as /smidʒli/, which would earn a score of 0.

   • *Item 17:* Student 1 shifts the vowel /o/ in "phonia" to "ah," saying /vopɪfɑniə/, thus earning a score of 0.

   • *Item 24:* Student 1 changes the vowel and substitutes a /p/ for /ɵ/, changing "transvathial" to "transvipial," scoring 0.

NW Rep

NONWORD REPETITION

Practice Items

Item	Actual/target spoken response
bup	bʌp /b ʌ p/

Item	Actual/target spoken response
stam	stæm /s t æ m/

Subtest Items

6–18

Item	Actual/target spoken response	Imitation score	
1. gid	/g ɪ d/	0	(1)
2. stenders	/s t ɛ n d ɚ z/ /s t ɪ n d ɚ z/	0	(1)
3. vilding	/v ɪ l d ɪ ŋ/	0	(1)
4. tep	/t ɛ p/	0	(1)
5. dabe	/d eɪ b/	0	(1)
6. tarbing	/t ɑr b ɪ ŋ/	0	(1)
7. skeap	/s k i p/	0	(1)
8. disvagle	/d ɪ s v eɪ g l̩/	0	(1)

Item	Actual/target spoken response	Imitation score	
9. glapped	/g l æ p t/	0	(1)
10. untigament	k /ʌ n t ɪ g ə m ɪ n t/ /ʌ n t ɪ g ə m ə n t/	(0)	1
11. scroil	skrɛl /s k r ɔɪ l/	(0)	1
12. droof	/d r u f/ /d r ʊ f/	0	(1)
13. interpidable	ɾ (flap)* /ɪ n t ɚ p ɪ d ə b l̩/	0	(1)
14. intosition	/ɪ n t o z ɪ ʃ ə n/	0	(1)
15. smitchly	/s m ɪ tʃ l i/	0	(1)
16. strenopious	/s t r ɛ n o p i ə s/ /s t r ɪ n o p i ə s/	0	(1)

Item	Actual/target spoken response	Imitation score	
17. vopiphonia	ah** /v o p ɪ f o n i ə/	(0)	1
18. mistudge	/m ɪ s t ʌ dʒ/	0	(1)
19. dopinician	/d o p ə n ɪ ʃ ə n/	0	(1)
20. nalted	/n ɔ l t ə d/ /n ɑ l t ə d/	0	(1)

Item	Actual/target spoken response	Imitation score	
21. nyvology	/n aɪ v ɑ l ə dʒ i/	0	(1)
22. vattle	/v æ t l/ [vocalic l̩] /v æ ɾ l/ [flap]	0	(1)
23. proderopia	/p r o d ɚ o p i ə/	0	(1)
24. transvathial	vipiəl /t r æ n z v eɪ θ i ə l/	(0)	1

Total score: 20 / 24

Qualitative observations:

*The flap is an articulatory variant of /d/ that counts as correct.
**Vowel shift might be counted correct if it were consistent with the child's regional dialect. In this case, it was not.

Nonword Repetition (NWRep) subtest scored for Student 1, a 6-year, 9-month-old boy.

SUBTEST 5: Nonword Spelling (NWSpell)

RECAP OF SUBTEST

In the Nonword Spelling (NWSpell) subtest, the student is asked to listen to nonwords presented on a digital recording and spell the words on the *TILLS Student Response Form*.

Use as a stand-alone measure: No (**Note:** Subtest 4 must be administered immediately prior to Subtest 5 and in the same session.)

Average time to administer: 6 minutes

Materials: *Examiner Record Form* (pp. 13–14), *Student Response Form* (p. 2), pencil with eraser, audio player, *Digital Audio Files* (Tracks 29–55)

Start rule: Start at the beginning for all students. (Do not administer Subtest 5 to children age 6;0–6;5.)

Basal rule: None

Ceiling rule: Scores 0 on 6 out of 8 consecutive items

Repetition: No (unless ambient noise interferes)

Probes: None

PRACTICE EXERCISE

The NWSpell subtest is scored using students' written responses on the *Student Response Form*. The first sample shows a *Student Response Form* completed by Student 1 (6-year, 9-month-old with normal language), and the second sample shows one completed by Student 2 (13-year-old with moderate-severe bilateral sensorineural hearing loss who uses binaural digital hearing aids). Score the students' responses using two blank *Examiner Record Forms*. Be sure to consider all allowable alternative spellings. Letter reversals or other orientation problems are counted as errors, but handwriting issues, such as failure to close letters, are not considered errors if they are consistent.

Ask yourself the following questions as you complete the exercise:

1. What must I do to establish a basal for the 6-year, 9-month-old student? For the 13-year-old student?

2. What must I do to establish a ceiling for these students?

3. What should I do if the student spells an item in a manner that seems acceptable but is not listed as an alternative on the *Examiner Record Form?*

4. Which responses in these two student examples should be counted as errors and scored 0?

5. What insights can I get from the NWSpell subtest into these two students' knowledge of how to map orthographic spellings onto the phonological and morphological structure of words? What evidence is provided by what they do well *and* what they miss?

ANSWERS

Make your best effort to complete the exercise before you read the following answers:

1. Start the voice recording at the beginning, with the two practice items first. Then, proceed with Item 1. This rule applies to students of any age (except students 6;0–6;5; do not administer this subtest for this age group). In other words, the basal on this subtest is always Item 1. Unlike administration of the NWRep subtest, when you can generally let the voice recording run, you may need to pause the recording after each NWSpell item to give the student time to spell it.

2. You should stop testing when the student scores 0 on 6 out of 8 consecutive items. This requires you to sit in a position where you can clearly see what the student is writing so you will know when to stop. If in doubt, it is better to test a few items beyond what you think might be the ceiling rather than to stop too soon. Any items spelled correctly above the ceiling must be given a score of 0, but it is better to have administered more than enough items than too few.

3. A student may spell an item in a manner that seems acceptable to you, but if it is not one of the acceptable alternatives on the *Examiner Record Form,* you must score the item 0. The reason for giving credit for alternative spellings only if they are listed on the *Examiner Record Form* is that the normative data are based on these scoring criteria.

4. The following commentary explains items of note for Student 1:

   - *Item 2:* Score 0 because the student writes "stend" for "stenders," omitting the final syllable (*-ers*), a common English morpheme but one that may be acquired later.

   - *Item 3:* Score 1 because the student writes the intended "vilding," which includes the final syllable (*-ing*), also a common English morpheme, and the bound morpheme that appears earliest in oral language. He also spells *-ing* correctly in the word "tarbing" (Item 6).

   - *Item 5:* Score 0 because the student spells "dabe" as "dae," omitting the final consonant sound but including the "silent *e*" that makes the medial vowel say the long *a* sound. He originally wrote "bae," but he spontaneously self-corrected (indicated by "sc" in scoring his response) the *b* to *d*. This effort could have led him to forget to represent the final /b/, but it is impossible to know that from observation alone.

   - *Item 8:* Score 1 because the student spells both the initial (*dis-*) and final (*-le*) morphemes correctly and also represents the "vag" consonant-vowel-consonant structure correctly in the middle syllable of "disvagle."

   - *Item 9:* Score 0 because the student's spelling of "glmt" for "glapped" has no vowel and the postvocalic phoneme /p/ is represented with *m* rather than with *p,* as in either of the correct options, "glapt" or "glapped."

   - *Items 10–14:* Score 0 because although the student shows unusual spelling knowledge for his age, he makes a variety of errors when attempting more complex phonemic, syllabic, and later-learned morphemic components.

   The following commentary explains items of note for Student 2:

   - *Item 2:* Score 1 because the student writes "stinders," for "stenders," which is one of the allowed alternatives.

   - *Item 9:* Score 1 because the student writes the intended response "glapped," which includes both the double consonants following the short vowel and the final morpheme *-ed.* This provides evidence that he is applying morphemic knowledge of the *-ed* ending, which is pronounced /t/ when it follows a voiceless sound (in this case, /p/). He would have earned credit for a phonetic spelling, "glapt," because it is analogous to the word "apt." However, if he had spelled the word as "glaped," the spelling would have earned 0 credit, because the single *p* would make the *a* a long vowel. Note that "glaped" also is not one of the listed alternatives.

   - *Item 10:* Score 0 because the student changes the "g" sound in the middle to a "v," perhaps due to speech perception difficulties related to his hearing loss.

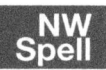

NONWORD SPELLING

- *Item 12:* Score 0 because the student spells "droof" as "druff," with a double consonant at the end. This changes the pronunciation of the vowel from /u/ to /ʌ/, and it is not one of the allowed alternatives.

- *Item 13:* Score 0 because the student's response of "intripidable" for "interpidable" is incorrect. Several alternatives are allowed for the initial morpheme (*inter-, intre-, intra-*), but "intri" is not one of them.

- *Item 16:* Score 0 because the student's spelling "shronophious" for "strenopious" is incorrect. This response involves using letters that represented phonemic substitutions: "sh" for /st/ and "ph" for /p/, which might reflect speech perception difficulties related to this student's hearing loss.

- *Item 17:* Score 1 because "vopophonia" is one of the accepted alternatives for "vopiphonia."

- *Item 18:* Score 0 because "mistoudge" is not one of the acceptable alternatives, even though it is reasonable.

- *Item 19:* Score 0 because "dirpinition" is not an acceptable alternative for "dopinition."

- *Item 20:* Score 0 because "naltid" is not one of the acceptable alternatives for "nalted."

- *Item 23:* Score 0 because "protorvppia" is not one of the acceptable alternatives. The long vowel /o/ called for a single *p* following.

- *Item 24:* Score 0 because the student substituted "p" for "th," changing the spelling of "transvathial" to "transvapial."

5. Responses on this subtest can provide insights into a student's knowledge of the phonological, orthographic, and morphological structures of words. Although Student 1 is young, he shows numerous areas of strength, consistent with his normal language development. He is reflective about his responses, so he takes longer than some of his same-age peers to complete this task. Several times he makes *b–d* reversals, but he self-corrects them. When asked about this later, he said that he was picturing the word *bed* to figure out which letter went with which sound. This child also shows emerging awareness of spelling of some morphemic components (*-ing* and *-le*). These abilities are consistent with his normal language development.

   Student 2 shows strengths in representing both the phonological and morphological structure of words, despite making some phonological errors that likely reflect speech perception difficulties related to his hearing loss. Noting these challenges, it is important for this student to see new vocabulary in print as well as hearing it in order to help him map the phonological structure accurately. His strengths included accurate spelling of several later-developing Latin- and Greek-influenced morphemes (e.g., *-ious, -phonia, -ology*). An area of inconsistency appeared in rules for using double consonants, which could be probed further in informal dynamic assessment following TILLS testing.

Practice Items

bop

ztam

Test Items

1. gia

2. stend

3. Vilding

4. tep

5. dae

6. tarbing

7. skeep

8. disvagle

9. glmt

10. utgumint

11. skral

12. grov

13. inthrpiabl

14. intosishin

15.

16.

17.

18.

19.

20.

21.

22.

23.

24.

Nonword Spelling (NWSpell) responses produced by Student 1,
a 6-year, 9-month-old boy.

Subtest Items

Item	Child's written response	Spelling score
6:6–18 → 1. gid	g i d	0 (1)
2. stenders	s t en d er s / in / z	(0) 1
3. vilding	v i l d ing / ui	0 (1)
4. tep	t e p	0 (1)
5. dabe	(sc) b- d a_e b (dabe)* / ai b / *(not daeb)	(0) 1
6. tarbing	t a r b ing	0 (1)

Item	Child's written response	Spelling score
7. skeap	s k ea p / ee / e_e (skepe)	0 (1)
8. disvagle	(sc) dis v a g le / f ei el / ai al	0 (1)
9. glapped	g l a m t pped / pt	(0) 1
10. untigament	u t g u / un t g a ment / i mant / mint	(0) 1
11. scroil	s k r a l / scr oi l / k oy al / le	(0) 1
12. droof	g r o v / d r oo f / u_e (drufe) / ou	(0) 1

(FORM PAGE BREAK)

Item	Child's written response	Spelling score
13. interpidable	inthr p i d bl / inter p i d able / intra t ible / intre tt	(0) 1
14. intosition	in t o z i shin / in t o s i tion / z sion / cian	(0) 1
15. smitchly	s m i tch ly / ch lie / ley	0 1
16. strenopious	s t r en o p ious / in ias / an ius / eous	0 1
17. vopiphonia	v o p i phonia / o fonia / a	0 1
18. mistudge	mis t u dge	0 1

ceiling

Item	Child's written response	Spelling score
19. dopinician	d o p i n i cian / a tion / o sion	0 1
20. nalted	n a l t ed / kn au / gn aw	0 1
21. nyvology	n y v ology / kn i	0 1
22. vattle	v a tt le / dd el	0 1
23. proderopia	pro d er o p ia / t or	0 1
24. transvathial	trans v a th ial / ai iel	0 1

Total score: 6 / 24

Qualitative observations:

Nonword Spelling (NWSpell) subtest scored for Student 1, a 6-year, 9-month-old boy.

NW Spell

NONWORD SPELLING

Practice Items

BUP

spom

Test Items

1. Gid
2. Stinders
3. Vilding
4. tep
5. Geb
6. Torbing
7. Skeep
8. disvagle
9. glopped
10. untivament
11. Skroil
12. druff

13. intripidable
14. intosition
15. Smitchly
16. Shronophious
17. Vopophonia
18. mistoudge
19. dirpinition
20. naltid
21. nivology
22. Vottle
23. protorveppia
24. transvopial

Nonword Spelling (NWSpell) responses produced by
Student 2, a 13-year-old boy. (*Note:* The scoring allowed for
a consistent pattern of how this student forms the letter *a*.)

Practice Items

Item	Child's written response
bup	b u p / b u p

Item	Child's written response
stam	s p a m / s t a m / mb

Subtest Items

Item	Child's written response	Spelling score		Item	Child's written response	Spelling score	
6;6–18 → 1. gid	g i d	0	(1)	7. skeap	s k ea p / ee / e_e (skepe)	0	(1)
2. stenders	s t en d er s / in z	0	(1)	8. disvagle	dis v a g le / f ei el / ai al	0	(1)
3. vilding	v i l d ing / ui	0	(1)	9. glapped	g l a pped / pt	0	(1)
4. tep	t e p	0	(1)	10. untigament	v / un t i g a ment / i mant / mint	(0)	1
5. dabe	g e b / d a_e b (dabe)* / ai b / *(not daeb)	(0)	1	11. scroil	s c r oi l / k oy al / le	0	(1)
6. tarbing	t a r b ing	0	(1)	12. droof	d r u ff / d r oo f / u_e (drufe) / ou	(0)	1

(FORM PAGE BREAK)

Item	Child's written response	Spelling score		Item	Child's written response	Spelling score	
13. interpidable	intri / inter p i d able / intra t ible / intre tt	(0)	1	19. dopinician	d ir / d o p i n i cian / a tion / o sion	(0)	1
14. intosition	in t o s i tion / z sion / cian	0	(1)	20. nalted	id / n a l t ed / kn au / gn aw	(0)	1
15. smitchly	s m i tch ly / ch lie / ley	0	(1)	21. nyvology	n y v ology / kn i	0	(1)
16. strenopious	sh r on o ph / s t r en o p ious / in ias / an ius / eous	(0)	1	22. vattle	v a tt le / dd el	0	(1)
17. vopiphonia	v o p i phonia / o fonia / a	0	(1)	23. proderopia	v pp / pro d er o p ia / t or	(0)	1
18. mistudge	mis t ou dge / mis t u dge	(0)	1	24. transvathial	p / trans v a th ial / ai iel	(0)	1

Total score: __14__ / 24

Qualitative observations:

Nonword Spelling (NWSpell) subtest scored for Student 2, a 13-year-old boy.

SUBTEST 6: Listening Comprehension (LC)

RECAP OF SUBTEST

In the Listening Comprehension (LC) subtest, the student is asked to listen to a one- to three-sentence "story" and answer questions with *yes, no,* or *maybe* based on information in the story.

Use as a stand-alone measure: Yes (**Note:** Subtest 6 can be used as a stand-alone measure or in conjunction with Subtest 7. If administered together with Subtest 7, Subtest 6 must be administered immediately before Subtest 7 and in the same session.)

Average time to administer: 7 minutes

Materials: *Examiner Record Form* (pp. 15–16)

Start rule: Start points for age ranges are indicated by arrows.

Basal rule: All 3 items correct for 2 consecutive stories

Ceiling rule: All 3 items incorrect for 2 consecutive stories

Repetition: No (except for practice story or if ambient noise interferes)

Probes: Yes (as specified in the *Examiner's Manual*)

PRACTICE EXERCISE

To complete this exercise, you will need to listen to Track 6 from the Examiner's Practice Workbook Audio Files folder on the *Digital Audio Files* (USB drive) for Student 1 and score the student's responses using a blank *Examiner Record Form*.

Ask yourself the following questions as you complete the exercise:

1. Which practice question is particularly important to prepare the student for this subtest?

2. The start point for Student 1 is Story 1. At what age should I begin with Story 2? What should I do if I start with Story 2 for a 15-year-old and the student gets all three questions correct but then misses Question A on Story 3?

3. How should I score the response to Question C on Story 3? Why?

4. Why does the examiner continue testing when Student 1 misses all 3 questions on Story 7?

ANSWERS

Make your best effort to complete the exercise before you read the following answers:

1. It is particularly important to explain to the student why the answer should be "maybe" for Question C on the practice story, which asks, "Does Teresa have a dog?" Coach the student to understand that the best answer is "maybe" because Teresa could have a dog; the story does not really tell us the answer.

2. Students age 12 years and older should begin with Story 2 after completing the practice story. If you start with Story 2 for a 15-year-old and the student gets all three questions correct for Story 2 but then misses Question A on Story 3, you should first finish Story 3. Then, back up and administer Story 1 to establish a basal. You can consider the basal established even if the student misses one or more of the questions on Story 1. Then, return to Story 4 and continue testing until you establish a ceiling.

3. Score the response to Question C on Story 3 as correct because the student self-corrects without any probing from the examiner.

4. Student 1 misses all 3 questions for Story 7, but the ceiling criterion is for the student to miss all 3 questions for 2 consecutive stories. This does not occur. Therefore, the examiner continues testing.

Teresa has a gray and white kitten that likes to play with string. The kitten's name is Fluffy.			
a. Is Teresa's kitten black?	Y	(N)	M
b. Does Teresa's kitten like to play with string?	(Y)	N	M
c. Does Teresa have a dog? *coach*	Y	(N) →	(M)

Subtest Items

1. The guy who makes the pizza crust can toss it in the air and catch it, but last night he had a little accident. He ended up with pizza dough hanging over his head.

a. Is the pizza maker always successful?	Y	(N)	M	0	(1)
b. Was he able to make some good crust last night?	Y	N	(M)	(0)	1
c. Did he ruin some crust last night?	(Y)	N	(M)	(0)	1

12+

2. Cassandra sat on the couch and got ready to watch the movie she liked best while her babysitter went into the kitchen to make popcorn. She had asked her babysitter to make cheese popcorn, but the babysitter brought back caramel popcorn instead. Cassandra exclaimed, "I didn't know you could make caramel popcorn. Caramel is my favorite!"

a. Did Cassandra help make popcorn?	Y	(N)	M	0	(1)
b. Was Cassandra getting ready to watch her favorite movie?	(Y)	N	M	0	(1)
c. Had Cassandra asked her babysitter to make caramel popcorn?	Y	(N)	M	0	(1)

3. The class did not understand the teacher's directions when she first told them how to complete the science project. When she showed them what to do step by step, however, the instructions made more sense.

a. Did all of the students understand the directions after the teacher's demonstration?	(Y)	N	(M)	(0)	1
b. Did the students know what to do at first?	Y	(N)	M	0	(1)
c. Did the class complete the assignment? *SC*	(Y)✗ → N	(M)	0	(1)

4. Immanuel was the first one of a small group of boys in his class who could dunk a basketball.

a. Could some of the other boys dunk a basketball?	(Y)	N	M	(0)	1
b. Could all of the boys in Immanuel's class dunk a basketball?	Y	(N)	M	0	(1)
c. Was Immanuel the best basketball player in the class?	Y	(N)	(M)	(0)	1

5. We thought it was strange that the art teacher told us to clean the brushes before we started painting. But when we realized that they really needed it, we followed his instructions.

a. Were the brushes dirty at first?	(Y)	N	M	0	(1)
b. Did we clean the brushes after we finished?	Y	(N)	(M)	(0)	1
c. Was the art teacher a woman?	Y	(N)	M	0	(1)

6. The land beyond the mountains was divided into two new territories. Each was to have its own governor, who would be selected by the President following consultation with his advisors.

a. Was a different governor going to be appointed for each new territory?	(Y)	N	M	0	(1)
b. Were the mountains part of the new territories?	Y	(N)	(M)	(0)	1
c. Was the President in charge of choosing the new governors?	(Y)	N	M	0	(1)

7. I asked Dan's sister why she was planning to take an umbrella to the beach. She said that if it rained, the umbrella would keep her dry, but if the sun was shining, it would protect her from the harmful rays.

a. Did Dan's sister forget her umbrella?	Y	(N)	(M)	(0)	1
b. Does Dan's sister think about things ahead of time?	(Y)	(N)	M	(0)	1
c. Did Dan's sister go alone to the beach?	Y	(N)	(M)	(0)	1

8. Mary and Todd decided they would go to the beach on Saturday even if it was a cloudy day. When they woke up on Saturday, it was sunny.

a. Did Mary and Todd plan to go to the beach on Saturday if it was cloudy?	(Y)	(N)	M	(0)	1
b. Did it rain later on Saturday?	Y	N	(M)	0	(1)
c. Was it cloudy when Mary and Todd woke up on Saturday?	Y	(N)	M	0	(1)

9. The scientists observed the insects closely over a 24-hour period, hoping to study their swarming behavior. At that point, the scientists concluded that the insects had been prevented from swarming because of the unusual atmospheric conditions.

a. Did the insects swarm during the observation period?	Y	(N)	(M)	(0)	1
b. Can atmospheric conditions influence the swarming of insects?	(Y)	N	M	0	(1)
c. Did the scientists accomplish their original goal?	Y	(N)	M	0	(1)

Total score: _15_ / 27

Qualitative observations:

Listening Comprehension (LC) subtest scored for Student 1, a 6-year, 9-month-old boy.

RECAP OF SUBTEST

In the Reading Comprehension (RC) subtest, the student is asked to read a one- to three-sentence story without assistance and answer questions with *yes, no,* or *maybe* based on information in the story.

Use as a stand-alone measure: No (*Note:* Subtest 6 must be administered immediately prior to Subtest 7 and in the same session.)

Average time to administer: 8 minutes

Materials: *Examiner Record Form* (pp. 17–18) *Student Response Form* (p. 3), pencil with eraser, cardstock (optional)

Start rule: Start points for age ranges are indicated by arrows. (Do not administer Subtest 7 to children age 6;0-6;5.)

Basal rule: All 3 questions correct for 2 consecutive stories

Ceiling rule: All 3 questions incorrect for 2 consecutive stories

Screening rule: Ask any student who might have a decoding problem to start by reading Story 1 aloud. If the student misreads seven or more words on the first story, discontinue testing, and write "emergent reader."

Repetition: Not applicable

Probes: Yes (as specified in the *Examiner's Manual*)

PRACTICE EXERCISE

To complete this exercise, you will need Track 7 from the Examiner's Practice Workbook Audio Files folder on the *TILLS Digital Audio Files* (USB drive) for Student 1, a 6-year, 9-month-old boy with normal language. The track is Student 1 reading Story 1 out loud. After Story 1, students may read subsequent stories either out loud or silently. Listen to the test administration on the audio file and mark any misread words on the blank *Examiner Record Form,* then complete the rest of the *Examiner Record Form* by referring to Student 1's responses on the *Student Response Form.*

Ask yourself the following questions as you complete the exercise:

1. Why is there no practice story for the RC subtest?

2. Why does the examiner ask the student to read Story 1 aloud? How many word errors does the student make when reading Story 1 aloud? What does this performance indicate about how to administer the rest of the test?

3. Under what circumstances should I stop the student from responding before completing all items on this subtest? That is, what is the ceiling rule?

ANSWERS

Make your best effort to complete the exercise before you read the following answers:

1. There is no practice story for this subtest because Listening Comprehension (LC) serves as practice. The two subtests use the same format, which is why it is essential to administer the LC subtest immediately prior to the RC subtest.

2. The examiner asked the student to read Story 1 aloud to ensure that his reading decoding skills were adequate to continue taking the subtest. The rule for making this decision is that the student must not misread seven or more words in order to proceed. Student 1 made errors on only four words ("my mother" for "a month," "give" for "gave," and "at least" for "usual"), so it was appropriate to continue. If he had misread seven or more words, the examiner would have ceased testing and assigned a score of 0 to this subtest. Hesitations, sounding out, and self-correction are not counted as errors in making this judgment, as this is not a reading fluency task.

3. You would stop the student from responding before completing all items on this subtest only if he missed all three questions for two consecutive stories (i.e., the ceiling rule).

1.	"What I Did on My Summer Vacation" is the topic the teacher makes her class write about the first day of school every year. When school started a month ago, the teacher gave her usual first writing assignment.			
a.	Was "The Middle East" the first writing assignment?	Yes	(No)	Maybe
b.	Did all of the students take a trip on their summer vacation?	Yes	No	(Maybe)
c.	Did the teacher ask her class to write about their summer vacations?	(Yes)	No	Maybe

2.	Last summer, Renaldo and Jake had fun in summer school learning new things. Photography was Renaldo's favorite class; in fact, the picture that Renaldo took of his friend Jake won the summer school prize.			
a.	Did Jake win the summer school prize?	(Yes)	No	Maybe
b.	Did Jake take a picture?	Yes	(No)	Maybe
c.	Did both boys have a good time in summer school?	Yes	No	(Maybe)

3.	Anna was excited when she thought about playing with her new hamster every day. However, she was surprised when she discovered that her hamster sleeps all day and runs on his wheel all night.			
a.	Does Anna's hamster sleep all night?	Yes	(No)	Maybe
b.	Did Anna expect her hamster to sleep all day before she brought him home?	Yes	No	(Maybe)
c.	Does Anna's hamster keep her awake all night?	Yes	No	(Maybe)

4.	All his friends thought that Carlos looked better before he had his hair cut by Juan.			
a.	Is Juan a barber?	Yes	No	(Maybe)
b.	Did Carlos's friends think Juan's haircut improved Carlos's looks?	Yes	(No)	Maybe
c.	Did Carlos like his new haircut?	(Yes)	No	Maybe

5.	One morning Susan got up too late to catch the school bus. She thought that she would be late for school, but her mother got her there on time.			
a.	Did Susan miss the bus?	(Yes)	No	Maybe
b.	Was it raining that morning?	Yes	No	(Maybe)
c.	Did Susan expect to miss the start of the school day?	Yes	(No)	Maybe

6.	The sport Eddie likes to play best is soccer. He can kick a soccer ball the second farthest in his class and run faster than anybody in his class.			
a.	Can Eddie kick a soccer ball farther than anyone else in his class?	(Yes)	No	Maybe
b.	Does Eddie like to play baseball?	Yes	No	(Maybe)
c.	Does Eddie run the fastest in his class?	(Yes)	No	Maybe

7.	The scientists observed the insects closely over a 24-hour period, hoping to study their swarming behavior. At that point, the scientists concluded that the insects had been prevented from swarming because of the unusual atmospheric conditions.			
a.	Did the insects swarm during the observation period?	(Yes)	No	Maybe
b.	Can atmospheric conditions influence the swarming of insects?	Yes	(No)	Maybe
c.	Did the scientists draw a conclusion even though the study did not go exactly as planned?	Yes	No	(Maybe)

Reading Comprehension (RC) subtest responses on the *Student Response Form* produced by Student 1, a 6-year, 9-month-old boy.

Subtest Items						

my mother   *give*   *at least*

6;6–11	1. "What I Did on My Summer Vacation" is the topic the teacher makes her class write about the first day of school every year. When school started [a month] ago, the teacher [gave] her [usual] first writing assignment.					
	a. Was "The Middle East" the first writing assignment?	Y	(N)	M	0	(1)
	b. Did all of the students take a trip on their summer vacation?	Y	N	(M)	0	(1)
	c. Did the teacher ask her class to write about their summer vacations?	(Y)	N	M	0	(1)

Read silently, following with eraser.

	2. Last summer, Renaldo and Jake had fun in summer school learning new things. Photography was Renaldo's favorite class; in fact, the picture that Renaldo took of his friend Jake won the summer school prize.					
	a. Did Jake win the summer school prize?	(Y)	(N)	M	(0)	1
	b. Did Jake take a picture?	Y	(N)	(M)	(0)	1
	c. Did both boys have a good time in summer school?	(Y)	N	(M)	(0)	1

12–14	3. Anna was excited when she thought about playing with her new hamster every day. However, she was surprised when she discovered that her hamster sleeps all day and runs on his wheel all night.					
	a. Does Anna's hamster sleep all night?	Y	(N)	M	0	(1)
	b. Did Anna expect her hamster to sleep all day before she brought him home?	Y	(N)	(M)	(0)	1
	c. Does Anna's hamster keep her awake all night?	Y	N	(M)	0	(1)

15+	4. All his friends thought that Carlos looked better before he had his hair cut by Juan.					
	a. Is Juan a barber?	Y	N	(M)	0	(1)
	b. Did Carlos's friends think Juan's haircut improved Carlos's looks?	Y	(N)	M	0	(1)
	c. Did Carlos like his new haircut?	(Y)	N	(M)	(0)	1

	5. One morning Susan got up too late to catch the school bus. She thought that she would be late for school, but her mother got her there on time.					
	a. Did Susan miss the bus?	(Y)	N	M	0	(1)
	b. Was it raining that morning?	Y	N	(M)	0	(1)
	c. Did Susan expect to miss the start of the school day?	(Y)	(N)	M	(0)	1

	6. The sport Eddie likes to play best is soccer. He can kick a soccer ball the second farthest in his class and run faster than anybody in his class.					
	a. Can Eddie kick a soccer ball farther than anyone else in his class?	(Y)	(N)	M	(0)	1
	b. Does Eddie like to play baseball?	Y	N	(M)	0	(1)
	c. Does Eddie run the fastest in his class?	(Y)	N	M	0	(1)

	7. The scientists observed the insects closely over a 24-hour period, hoping to study their swarming behavior. At that point, the scientists concluded that the insects had been prevented from swarming because of the unusual atmospheric conditions.					
	a. Did the insects swarm during the observation period?	(Y)	(N)	M	(0)	1
	b. Can atmospheric conditions influence the swarming of insects?	(Y)	(N)	M	(0)	1
	c. Did the scientists draw a conclusion even though the study did not go exactly as planned?	(Y)	N	(M)	(0)	1

Total score: _11_ / 21

Qualitative observations:

Place a checkmark beside strategies observed:

√ Moving the card from line to line

√ Scanning left to right

√ Looking back to the story

Other: This student was very systematic in reading and checking his answers. Unusual for a child his age.

Reading Comprehension (RC) subtest scored for Student 1, a 6-year, 9-month-old boy.

RECAP OF SUBTEST

In the Following Directions (FD) subtest, the examiner covers the visual stimuli in the *Student Response Form* with cardstock. The student is asked to listen to oral directions that involve using a pencil to perform such actions as to circle, cross out, and underline shapes, numbers, and letters. The student will then uncover the visual stimuli and follow the directions by writing in the *Student Response Form* with a pencil.

Use as a stand-alone measure: Yes	**Basal rule:** 6 consecutive scores of 1
Average time to administer: 8 minutes	**Ceiling rule:** Scores 0 on 6 out of 8 consecutive items
Materials: *Examiner Record Form* (pp. 19–20), *Student Response Form* (pp. 4–6), pencil with eraser, cardstock	**Repetition:** No (unless ambient noise interferes)
	Probes: None
Start rule: Start points for age ranges are indicated by arrows	

PRACTICE EXERCISE

This subtest must be scored while observing the student respond to spoken directions by marking the *Student Response Form* with a pencil. Direct observation is essential for items that specify a particular sequence or direction. In addition, for these and other items, you should check your scoring against the paper-and-pencil record produced by the student. To complete this exercise, look at the *Student Response Form* completed by Student 1, a 6-year, 9-month-old boy, and score any responses that you can using a blank *Examiner Record Form*. Then, look at the examiner's representation of the student's responses and check the examiner's notes about directionality (shown with arrows) and sequence (actions numbered 1, 2, 3).

Ask yourself the following questions as you complete the exercise:

1. Student 1 begins with Item 1. At what ages should I begin testing with higher numbered items?

2. Which items can I score by looking at the student's responses? Which items require reference to the examiner's notes?

3. Why does the examiner stop testing with Item 16?

ANSWERS

Make your best effort to complete the exercise before you read the following answers:

1. Testing begins with Item 1 for students age 6–9 years. For students age 10–14 years, testing begins with Item 5. For students age 15 years and above, testing begins with Item 10. If a student starts at one of these higher start points but then fails to reach the basal criterion of six consecutive items correct, it is essential to test backward from the start point to establish a basal. Testing backward begins with the item immediately previous to the designated starting item and proceeds in a "countdown" manner to previous items until the basal is met or Item 1 has been administered.

2. Any items that do not specify a line direction (*from* x *to* y) or a sequence ("before," "after," "then," etc., marked with the word "[Sequence]") can be scored by looking at the student's completed responses. All other items require reference to the examiner's notes. You may note that the examiner numbers sequence on some items where it is not required. Doing so is not essential, but it ensures the numbers will be there if needed.

3. When Student 1 makes an error on Item 16 that meets the criterion of 0 on 6 out of 8 consecutive items for the ceiling on this subtest, so testing stops.

Practice Items

Test Items

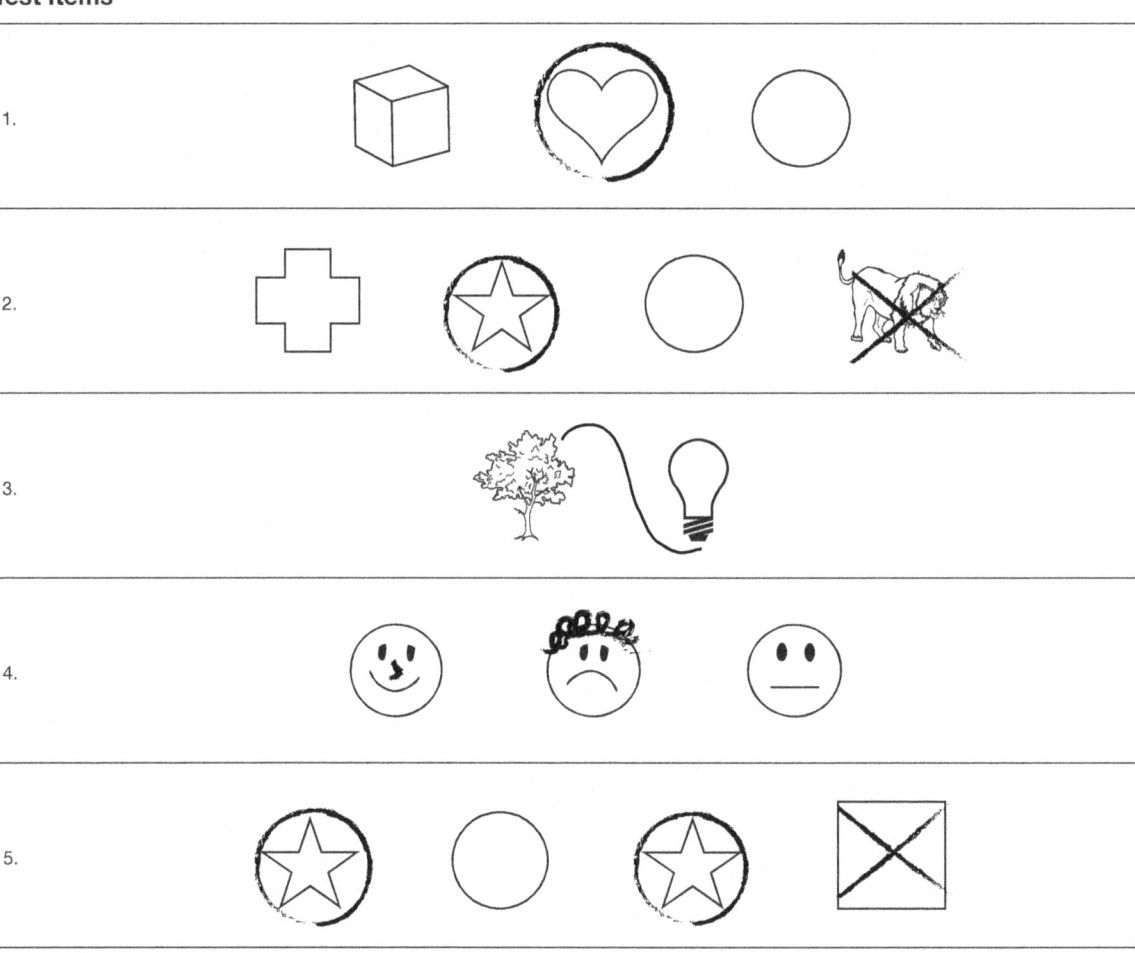

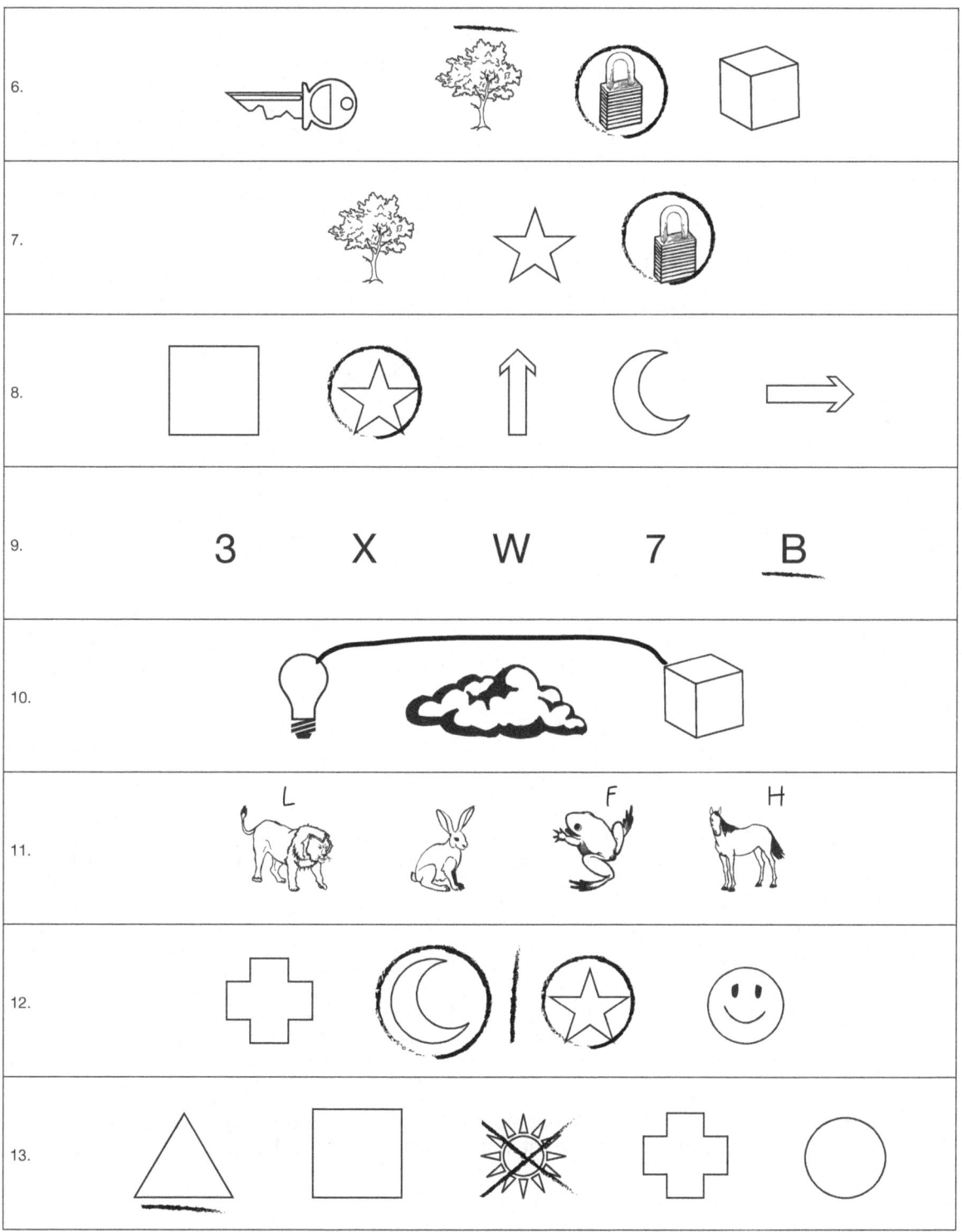

14.					

15.					

16.				

17.			

18.				

19.	E	88	e	20	S	16

20.	2	f	a	C	F

Following Directions (FD) subtest responses on the *Student Response Form* produced by Student 1, a 6-year, 9-month-old boy.

Practice Items

Instructions	Student's response (from *Student Response Form*)
Number 1: Cross out the circle. Go. [Either an X or single line may be used to "cross out."]	
Number 2: Draw an arrow from the heart to the box. Go.	

Subtest Items

	Instructions	Student's response (from *Student Response Form*)	Score	
6–9	Number 1: Draw a circle around the heart. Go.		0	(1)
	Number 2: Cross out the lion and circle the star. Go. [Either an X or single line may be used to "cross out."]		0	(1)
	Number 3: Draw a line from the top of the tree to the bottom of the light bulb. Go.		0	(1)
	Number 4: Draw hair on the sad face and put a nose on the happy face. Go.		0	(1)
10–14	Number 5: When you have finished circling all the stars, cross out the square. Go. [Sequence] [Say, **"Turn the page."**]		0	(1)
	Number 6: Draw a line above the tree and circle the lock. Go. [Line may be horizontal or vertical.]		0	(1)
	Number 7: If the lock is in the middle, underline the star. If not, circle the tree. Go.		(0)	1
	Number 8: If there is an arrow pointing down, draw a circle under the moon. If not, circle the star. Go.		0	(1)
	Number 9: If there is a number 3, underline the B. If not, circle the X. Go.		0	(1)
15+	Number 10: Before you cross out the cloud, draw an arrow from the light bulb over the cloud to the box. Go. [Sequence] [Line through the cloud does not count]		(0)	1
	Number 11: Write a letter F above the frog, an L above the lion, and then an H above the horse. Go. [Lowercase is acceptable.] [Sequence]		(0)	1
	Number 12: Circle the star then the moon, but before that, draw a line between them. Go. [Line may be horizontal or vertical.] [Sequence]		0	(1)
	Number 13: Before you cross out the sun, underline the triangle and then the cross. Go. [Sequence] [Say, **"Turn the page."**]		(0)	1
	Number 14: Write a number 1 in the first shape on the left, a 2 in the center shape, and a 3 in the last shape on the right. Cross out the other 2 shapes. Go.		(0)	1

Number 15: Write a letter S in the circle in the middle, cross out the S that is inside the square, and circle the S that is outside the square. Go.		(0)	1
Number 16: After you give the happy face a nose, put a dot in the center of the triangle and the cross. Then underline the star. Go. [Sequence]		(0)	1
Number 17: Start by circling the books. Then draw a line from the top of the books under the tree and into the center of the star. Go. [Sequence]		0	1 *ceiling*
Number 18: Draw a line from the lightning bolt over the moon and into the sun. Then draw a circle under the arrow. Go. [Sequence] [Line through moon does not count.]		0	1
Number 19: Cross out the largest number and draw a line from the lowercase e to the S over the number between them. Go.		0	1
Number 20: Underline both Fs. Draw a line over the 2, and cross out the A. Go. [Line over the 2 may be horizontal or vertical.]		0	1

Total score: 9 / 20

Qualitative observations:

Following Directions (FD) subtest scored for a 6-year, 9-month-old boy.

RECAP OF SUBTEST

In the Delayed Story Retelling (DSR) subtest, the student is asked to retell the same story heard 20–30 minutes previously without hearing it again.

Use as a stand-alone measure: No (*Note:* Subtest 9 must be administered 20–30 minutes following Subtest 3, with language-related activities intervening.)

Average time to administer: 2 minutes

Materials: *Examiner Record Form* (pp. 21–22), audio recording device (recommended)

Story A: "Tommy the Trickster" for ages 6;0–11;11 (p. 7 of the *Examiner Record Form*)

Story B: "The Rubber Raft" for ages 12;0–18;11 (p. 9 of the *Examiner Record Form*)

Start rule: Arrows with age ranges in years indicate which story to administer.

Basal rule: None

Ceiling rule: None

Repetition: Not applicable

Probes: Yes (as specified in the *Examiner's Manual*)

PRACTICE EXERCISE

To complete this exercise, you will need Track 8 from the Examiner's Practice Workbook Audio Files folder on the *Digital Audio Files* (USB drive) for Student 1, a 6-year, 9-month-old boy with normal language, and Track 9 for Student 2, a 13-year-old boy with moderate-severe bilateral sensorineural hearing loss who uses binaural digital hearing aids. Listen to the test administration on the audio file. Score Student 1's responses to Story A and Student 2's responses to Story B using a blank *Examiner Record Form.* As for Story Retelling (SR), listen to each story more than once to confirm scoring.

Ask yourself the following questions as you complete the exercise:

1. Which items are most challenging to score for Stories A and B?

2. How do the students' responses for this subtest compare with their original responses for Story Retelling (SR)?

ANSWERS

Make your best effort to complete the exercise before you read the following answers:

1. Scoring for Student 1 is fairly straightforward; however, he makes a few changes in wording that make scoring a bit challenging. At the beginning, he says, "Tommy was a fat boy," earning credit for Items 1 and 4. At that point, however, he says, "His mother worried about him." The examiner gives credit for Items 2 and 3 because "worried" captures the essence of his mother's mental state, "thought." The student also earns credit for telling how Tommy traded his healthy foods for his friends' cookies. Although he never mentions "friends" (so he does not get credit for Item 20), he uses direct quotes to act out the conversation about trading. Thus, he receives credit for Items 18–24, with the exception of Item 20.

   Scoring for Student 2 is similar to scoring his initial retelling. He uses the name "Angela," which is a form of "Angie," at the beginning of the story, so it receives credit. He still cannot remember what the activity "director" (for "leader") had asked the pair to do, but he does say, "He asked them to do something," for which he earns credit for Content Unit 14 ("he said"). As in the original retelling, he says, "they got something to drink" to earn credit for Content Unit 31 and says, "when they came back" to earn credit for Content Units 32 and 33, "as (while/when) they were walking back." This time, when he reaches the end of the story, he first uses the word "plastic" to refer to the deflated raft but then shifts to "rubber," which was the term used in the original story.

2. Student 1 does an interesting thing before initiating his delayed retelling. When the examiner prompts him to begin retelling the story, he says, "I'm thinking about it." Then, he rehearses his entire retelling subvocally, demonstrating unusual executive skills for a 6-year-old. He incorporates almost as many content units in the retold story (20 of the 33) as in the original retelling (24 of the 33).

Student 2 also scores similarly on the Story Retelling (SR) and Delayed Story Retelling (DSR) subtests, earning 32 of 51 points on the SR subtest and 33 of 51 points on the DSR subtest. This indicates that he has strong story comprehension, memory, and executive function abilities. In addition, shifting from the word "plastic" to "rubber" after hearing the word in the comprehension questions following the SR subtest is a positive prognostic indicator for this student's language learning ability.

Content Units		Score		Content Units		Score	
1. Tommy's (must use proper name to count on first instance)	0	(1)		18. at school	0	(1)	
2. mother	0	(1)		19. he convinced (talked them into, told)	0	(1)	
3. thought he (Tommy, worried)	(0)	1		20. his friends	(0)	1	
4. was getting fat (bigger, gaining weight)	0	(1)		21. that cookies	0	(1)	
5. from eating	0	1		22. were bad	0	(1)	
6. too much	0	1		23. for them	0	(1)	
7. junk food (cookies)	0	1		24. then he traded	0	(1)	
8. so she	0	(1)		25. his fruit (healthy foods [only scores once])	(0)	1	
9. stocked (put)	0	(1)		26. carrots (carrot sticks, healthy foods) *veg & car*	0	(1)	
10. the refrigerator (fridge, icebox)	0	(1)		27. for cookies	0	(1)	
11. fruit (healthy foods [only scores once] [not grapes, etc.*])	(0)	1		28. his mother	0	(1)	
12. carrots (carrot sticks, healthy foods, vegetables)	0	(1)		29. didn't know why	0	(1)	
13. she even put	0	1		30. Tommy (he)	0	(1)	
14. these things	0	1		31. kept gaining weight (getting bigger/fatter)	0	(1)	
15. in his lunchbox (lunch bag, lunch)	0	1		32. when all she had given him	(0)	1	
16. but Tommy (he)	0	(1)		33. were healthy foods *ran*	(0)	1	
17. was a "fast talker" (figurative meaning)	(0)	1					

*The scoring guideline is that a child can get credit for a superordinate category label (*vegetables* for *carrots*) but not a more specific one (e.g., *grapes* for *fruit* does not earn credit).

Total score: 20 / 33

Qualitative observations:

Delayed Story Retelling (DSR) subtest (Story A) scored for Student 1, a 6-year, 9-month-old boy.

Content Units	Score	
1. (last) summer	(0)	1
2. Michael (must use proper name)	0	(1)
3. Angie (must use proper name) Angela	0	(1)
4. went	0	(1)
5. to the lake (beach)	0	(1)
6. at the park	0	(1)
7. when they got there	(0)	1
8. they asked	0	(1)
9. activity	0	(1)
10. leader (accept synonyms [only score once]) director	0	(1)
11. if they could use borrow	0	(1)
12. one	(0)	1
13. of the rubber rafts	0	(1)
14. he said he asked them to do something	0	(1)
15. they could (yes)	0	1
16. if they would	0	1
17. pump it up (blow it up, inflate it)	0	1
18. by the time	0	(1)
19. they finished got done	0	(1)
20. inflating (pumping up, blowing it up)	0	(1)
21. the raft (rubber boat, rubber thing)	0	(1)
22. Michael (the kids/they [only scores once])	(0)	1
23. Angie (the kids)	0	(1)
24. were tired	0	(1)
25. and thirsty	0	(1)
26. so they left	(0)	1

Content Units	Score	
27. the raft	0	1
28. by the lake	0	1
29. while they went	0	1
30. to the snack bar	0	1
31. for a drink they got something to drink	0	(1)
32. as (while/when) when	0	(1)
33. they were walking back they came back	0	(1)
34. they spotted (saw)	(0)	1
35. a huge (large)	0	1
36. gray	0	(1)
37. cat	0	(1)
38. with claws out	(0)	1
39. getting ready	0	(1)
40. to pounce	0	(1)
41. on the raft	0	(1)
42. they started running ran	0	(1)
43. toward the raft	0	(1)
44. yelling at	(0)	1
45. the cat	0	1
46. (but) by the time (when)	0	(1)
47. they got there	0	(1)
48. it was too late	(0)	1
49. they were looking at looked like	0	(1)
50. a rubber plastic → rubber	0	(1)
51. pancake	0	(1)

Total score: 33 / 51

DSR

Qualitative observations:

Delayed Story Retelling (DSR) subtest (Story B) scored for Student 2, a 13-year-old boy.

RECAP OF SUBTEST

In the Nonword Reading (NWRead) subtest, the student is asked to read "pretend words" aloud one at a time from a list in the *Stimulus Book* as an assessment of reading decoding.

Use as a stand-alone measure: Yes

Average time to administer: 4 minutes

Materials: *Examiner Record Form* (pp. 23–24), *Stimulus Book* (pp. 57–67), audio recording device (recommended)

Start rule: Start points for age ranges are indicated by arrows. (Do not administer to children age 6;0–6;5.)

Basal rule: 6 consecutive scores of 1

Ceiling rule: Scores 0 on 6 out of 8 consecutive items

Repetition: Not applicable

Probes: Yes (as specified in the *Examiner's Manual*)

PRACTICE EXERCISE

To complete this exercise, you will need Track 10 from the Examiner's Practice Workbook Audio Files folder on the *Digital Audio Files* (USB drive) for Student 1, a 6-year, 9-month-old boy with normal language. Listen to the test administration on the audio file and score Student 1's responses using a blank *Examiner Record Form*. Note that target spoken responses for this subtest are presented using IPA symbols; however, it is acceptable to record differences in the student's response from the target correct response using standard orthography or by marking changes, such as substituted, inserted, or deleted phonemes, on either the orthographic spelling or phonetic representation in the *Examiner Record Form*. As with the Nonword Repetition (NWRep) subtest, it is important to have good phonemic awareness skills to administer and score this test, but it is not necessary to know the IPA.

Ask yourself the following questions as you complete the exercise:

1. The examiner starts with Item 1. How would this differ if the student were 8 years old and made an error on the third item administered?

2. When is the ceiling established?

3. Which items provide information that is helpful for understanding this student's decoding abilities?

4. Observe the parallel structure in these nonword items to items that appear in Nonword Repetition (NWRep) and Nonword Spelling (NWSpell). How might I use this structure to understand more about a student's strengths and weaknesses?

ANSWERS

Make your best effort to complete the exercise before you read the following answers:

1. Testing starts with Item 1 for 6;6- to 7-year-olds (p. 59 in the *Stimulus Book*). Other start points are specified for older students, always beginning with the first item on a page in the *Stimulus Book*. Students who are age 8–10 years start with Item 4, "dape" (p. 61); students age 11–13 years start with Item 7, "mistation" (p. 63); and students age 14 and older start with Item 11, "shreebing" (p. 65). Whether testing forward to the ceiling or backward to establish a basal, always start with the top item on a page. If the student makes errors before establishing a basal and you must turn to a prior page, begin at the top of the page and test to

the bottom to ensure that the basal is established and all items above the basal have been administered.

2. The criterion for the ceiling is scoring 0 on 6 out of 8 consecutive items. Student 1 reaches the ceiling on Item 18, based on missing Items 10, 13, 14, 15, 16, and 17. He scores 0 on Item 18, but even if he had passed it, the examiner would have had to score it as 0 because it is above the ceiling.

3. Student 1 demonstrates language and literacy strengths as well as some developmentally appropriate errors. Items of interest include the following:

   • *Item 1:* Score 1 because the student correctly reads the middle vowel in "pog" as /ɑ/, demonstrating awareness of the effect of the consonant-vowel-consonant on pronunciation of the medial vowel when no final *e* is present.

   • *Item 2:* Score 1 because the student first reads "keb" as "kep," but then he self-corrects, changing the final consonant from /kɛp/ to /kɛb/.

   • *Item 3:* Score 0 because the student inserts a schwa vowel in the initial consonant cluster in "troom" and then reads the double "oo" vowel as /o/ rather than /u/, pronouncing the word as /tərom/ rather than /trum/.

   • *Item 4:* Score 1 because the student demonstrates the ability to map the orthographic pattern for long vowel plus silent *e* by saying "dabe."

   • *Item 5:* Score 1 because the student demonstrates correct mapping of orthographic and morphemic patterns to phonology by saying "glenders."

   • *Item 6:* Score 0 because the student demonstrates difficulty with the diphthong /ɔɪ/ in "sproil," inserting another /l/ in the middle and pronouncing it as "spralil."

   • *Item 7:* Score 0 because the student does not read the final morpheme "tion" as /ʃən/ (pronounced "shun"); rather, he reads the initial sound as /t/. The *-tion* morpheme is somewhat later developing than *-ing*, which is a morpheme he reads correctly two times (in Items 11 and 12).

   • *Items 8–9:* Score 1 for each because the student represents the phonological and morphological components of these two words, "stig" and "shiggle," correctly in his spoken responses.

   • *Item 10:* Score 0 because by saying /bræpɛld/ for "brapped," the student shows incomplete or missing knowledge of the rule for pronouncing the final *-ed* morpheme as /t/ when it occurs following a voiceless consonant (in this case /p/).

   • *Items 11–12:* Score 1 for each because the student demonstrates knowledge of how to pronounce the final *-ing* morpheme in both these words and also reads the stems of both words correctly.

   • *Item 13:* Score 0 because the student omits the nasal /n/ from his reading of "unverly" but otherwise reads this word correctly. Still, the omission leads to a score of 0 on the item.

   • *Items 14–17:* Score 0 because the student demonstrates a phonetic approach to attempting to read the orthographic patterns. For these more complex words, he does not seem to be using information about common morphemes, including the *-ed,* which gives him difficulty on Item 10 as well as Item 14, and he shows no awareness of later developing morphemes, such as *-ology.* He would not be expected to have knowledge of Greek orthographic elements, given his 6-year, 9-month-old age.

4. When a student responds to orthographic patterns in one modality, such as in Nonword Reading (NWRead), those responses can be compared to how the student responds to similar phonological and orthographic patterns on the Nonword Repetition (NWRep) and Nonword Spelling (NWSpell) tasks (Subtests 4 and 5). It is interesting to note that Student 1 demonstrates similar morphemic knowledge on the NWRead and NWSpell tasks, with consistent awareness of the *-ing* morpheme and how it is read (on "shreebing" and "tilding" among the NWRead items), as well as how it is pronounced and spelled (on "vilding" and "tarbing" among the NWRep and NWSpell items), earning scores of 1 on all of these items. Parallel findings also are indicated by responses to the NWRead and NWSpell subtests that show that knowledge of other morphemes is still emerging, as one would expect for a student of this age.

Subtest Items

Stimulus word	Expected production (and acceptable alternatives)	Score		Stimulus word	Expected production (and acceptable alternatives)	Score
6;6–7 1. pog	———— /pɔg/ /pɑg/	0 (1)	**11–13**	7. mistation	mıstaɛtian /mɪs teˈ ʃən/	(0) 1
2. keb	kɛp (SC) /kɛb/	(0̷) (1)		8. steeg	———— /stig/	0 (1)
3. troom [Turn the page.]	tərom /trum/	(0) 1		9. shiggle	———— /ʃɪˈ gl̩/	0 (1)
8–10 4. dape	———— /dēɪp/	0 (1)		10. brapped [Turn the page.]	bræpɛld /bræpt/	(0) 1
5. glenders	———— /glɛnˈ dɚz/ /glɪnˈ dɚz/	0 (1)	**14+**	11. shreebing	———— /ʃriˈ bɪŋ/	0 (1)
6. sproil [Turn the page.]	spralɪl /sprɔ̄ɪl/	(0) 1		12. tilding	———— /tɪlˈ dɪŋ/	0 (1)

(FORM PAGE BREAK)

Stimulus word	Expected production (and acceptable alternatives)	Score	Stimulus word	Expected production (and acceptable alternatives)	Score
13. unverly	~~ɤ~~ /ʌnˈ vɚ li/ /ʌn vɚˈ li/	(0) 1	19. redikament	———— /ri dɪ kə mɪnt/	0 1
14. ralted	rælɪtɪn /rɔlˈ təd/	(0) 1	20. nopiphonia	———— /no pɪ foˈ ni ə/ /nɑ pɪ foˈ ni ə/	0 1
15. distudge	diʃtɪgɛ /dɪs tʌʤ/	(0) 1	21. interdepable	———— /ɪn tɚ dɛpˈ əbl̩/	0 1
16. gorentobia	garɪntabɪæ /go rən toˈ bi ə/ /go rɛn toˈ bi ə/	(0) 1	22. smorifious	———— /smor ɪˈ fi əs/ /smor ɪ fiˈ əs/	0 1
17. plitchly	plɪtʃi /plɪtʃ̷ li/	(0) 1	23. periothial	———— /per i ɑˈ θi əl/ /per i oˈ θi əl/ /per i o θiˈ əl/	0 1
18. tyvology [Turn the page.]	*teɪvalági /taɪv aˈ lə ʤi/	(0) 1	24. kizmanician	———— /kɪz mə nɪˈ ʃən/	0 1

ceiling

Total score: __8__ / 24

Qualitative observations:

*Score as 0 regardless of student's performance because this item is above the ceiling.

Nonword Reading (NWRead) subtest scored for Student 1, a 6-year, 9-month-old boy.

RECAP OF SUBTEST

In the Reading Fluency (RF) subtest, the student is asked to read real words in short sentences from a list of "facts" in an age-appropriate story as an assessment of automatic word recognition and reading fluency.

Use as a stand-alone measure: Yes (*Note:* Subtest 11 can be used as a stand-alone measure or in conjunction with Subtest 12. If administered together with Subtest 12, Subtest 11 must be administered immediately before Subtest 11 and in the same session.)

Average time to administer: 2 minutes

Materials: *Examiner Record Form* (pp. 25–28), *Stimulus Book* (correct story for age), audio recording device (recommended)

Start rule: Arrows with age ranges in years indicate which story to administer. (Do no administer Subtest 11 to children age 6;0–6;5.)

Story A: "The Class Pet" for ages 6;6–7;11 (p. 69)

Story B: "The Principal's Daughter" for ages 8;0–10;11 (p. 71)

Story C: "When the School Closed" for ages 11;0–13;11 (p. 73)

Story D: "The Building" for ages 14;0–18;11 (p. 75)

Basal rule: None

Ceiling rule: If the student becomes upset or anxious, you may decide to discontinue. If so, count any unread words as 0.

Repetition: Not applicable

Probes: Yes (as specified in the *Examiner's Manual*)

PRACTICE EXERCISE

To complete this exercise, you will need Track 11 from the Examiner's Practice Workbook Audio Files folder on the *Digital Audio Files* (USB drive) for Student 1, a 6-year, 9-month-old boy with normal language. Listen to the test administration on the audio file and score Student 1's responses using a blank *Examiner Record Form*. Note that fluent reading on the TILLS is defined as reading words in context without unusual pausing or hesitation and without repeating words or phrases or making any changes in the words printed on the page. If the student repeats more than one word, you should subtract only 1 because it may be hesitation over how to read the upcoming word that led to the repetition, even though the student repeats a whole phrase. If a student inserts a word that is not present in the print, subtract 1 point from the total for that line.

Ask yourself the following questions as you complete the exercise:

1. What are the basal and ceiling rules? What must I do if I administer the wrong story for the student's age by mistake? Are there different rules for which story to use when testing students with severe language and literacy impairments or students with intellectual developmental disabilities?

2. The first thing the examiner asks the student to do on this subtest is to read the title of the age-appropriate story out loud. What should I do if a student struggles to read the title or reads words in the title incorrectly? Is it acceptable to help students sound out words or tell them words they cannot read on this subtest?

3. Does the student earn credit if he or she self-corrects a word?

4. Which items on this subtest are most challenging to score? Why?

ANSWERS

Make your best effort to complete the exercise before you read the following answers:

1. There are no basal or ceiling rules for this subtest. All students are encouraged to attempt all items in their age-appropriate story. Failure to administer the correct

story for the student's age is the most common error examiners make in administering the Reading Fluency (RF) and Written Expression (WE) subtests. If you should make this error and not notice it until after you end the session, you must reschedule the student for another session and then administer the correct story for the student's age. This is the only way you can compare the student's scores to normative data. *There are no exceptions!* Students with severe language and literacy disorders or with intellectual developmental disabilities must be administered stories appropriate to their chronological age if the examiner wishes to compare these students' scores to the normative data.

2. The purpose of having students read the title of their story out loud before proceeding to read the facts is to orient them to the task. In addition, this can give you an idea of how difficult this subtest is likely to be for the student. If a student struggles to read the title, encourage him or her to attempt all of the items on this subtest, but use the probe "Just read the words you know." It is absolutely *not* acceptable to help students sound out words or tell them words they cannot decode. Doing so invalidates the remainder of this subtest. If students express frustration with this subtest, encourage them to read only the words they know. If that does not help, stop testing and assign scores of 0 to any remaining items. You will be able to read the facts aloud to a student who had difficulty reading them independently immediately prior to administering the Written Expression (WE) subtest.

3. This subtest measures reading fluency, not decoding accuracy, so if a student self-corrects a word, he or she is not reading fluently. Self-corrected words score 0, reducing the total possible item score by 1.

4. The fluency errors made by Student 1 follow:

   - *Item 3:* The student pauses before the word "spots," which means that he earns a 0 for this word, and 3 out of the possible score of 4 for the four-word sentence "The hamster has spots." Then, he misreads the word "spots" as "stops," but this does not change the item score of 3 because he already has been penalized for not reading the word "spots" fluently. Early readers may use a one-word-at-a-time reading prosody (rhythm) rather than using natural phrasing. This cadence should not be penalized as long as the rhythm is steady and their pauses are under 1 second. If students read in this manner, you can make note of this under Qualitative Observations.

   - *Item 8:* The student initially reads "change" for "cage" but then self-corrects the error. Even so, he scores 0 on that word, earning a score of 3 out of 4 on this item. Remember, this subtest assesses reading fluency plus accuracy, not reading accuracy alone, so self-corrected words still count as 0 on this subtest.

   - *Item 13:* The student fluently misreads "the" as "his" in the sentence "They put him in the cage." The substituted word fits the context, but it still counts as an error because words must be read both fluently and accurately. Thus, the student earns a score of 5 out of 6 on this item.

   - *Item 15:* The student hesitates prior to the phrase "a corner." Only 1 point is deducted rather than 2 for the hesitation on this phrase, or for the repetition of any phrase, because the fluency glitch can generally be attributed to one problematic word. After a short pause to allow this student to attempt to decode "corner," the examiner prompts the student to move on and just read the words he knows.

READING FLUENCY SCORING FORM
Story A: "The Class Pet" (p. 69)

Story elements	Score	Story elements	Score
Title: The Class Pet	3 /3	9. The door was open.	4 /4
1. The class has a pet.	5 /5	10. The children looked.	3 /3
2. It is a hamster.	4 /4	11. The children found him.	4 /4
pause–stops 3. The hamster has spots.	③ /4	12. They put him back.	4 /4
4. Some are brown.	3 /3	*his* / *fluent misreading* 13. They put him in the cage.	⑤ /6
5. Some are white.	3 /3	14. They closed the door.	4 /4
6. It got out.	3 /3	*hesitate K – unable to decode corner* *Note: prompt to move on* 15. He found a corner.	③ /4
7. It was one day last week.	6 /6	16. He went to sleep.	4 /4
change SC / *misreading followed by self-correction* 8. The cage was open.	③ /4	Column total	31 /33
	Column total 33 /35	Total score	64 /68

Qualitative observations:

Note: Child mentioned having a class pet. Examiner (eventually) responded to this spontaneous comment, but avoided the word "hamster"

*Child hesitated prior to "a corner" on item 15. When the child hesitates prior to a phrase or repeats the whole phrase, only one word error is counted unless the child misreads both words.

Reading Fluency (RF) subtest scored for Student 1, a 6-year, 9-month-old boy.

RECAP OF SUBTEST

The Written Expression (WE) subtest should be administered immediately after the Reading Fluency (RF) subtest. The student is shown "The Little Dog" on page 77 of the *Stimulus Book*. Then, the student is shown how the facts are rewritten on page 7 of the *Student Response Form*. The student is asked to rewrite the facts from his or her story so that they sound less choppy and more interesting.

Use as a stand-alone measure: No (*Note:* Subtest 11 must be administered immediately prior to Subtest 12 and in the same session.)

Average time to administer: 10 minutes

Materials: *Examiner Record Form* (pp. 29–31), *Stimulus Book* (p. 77; then correct story for age), *Student Response Form* (pp. 7–8)

Start rule: Arrows with age ranges in years indicate which story to administer. (Do not administer Subtest 12 to children age 6;0-6;5.)

Story A: "The Class Pet" for ages 6;6–7;11 (p. 69)

Story B: "The Principal's Daughter" for ages 8;0–10;11 (p. 71)

Story C: "When the School Closed" for ages 11;0–13;11 (p. 73)

Story D: "The Building" for ages 14;0–18;11 (p. 75)

Basal rule: None

Ceiling rule: If the student indicates being finished, record the time spent writing and move to the next subtest

Repetition: Not applicable

Probes: Yes (as specified in the *Examiner's Manual*)

PRACTICE EXERCISE

If you are uncertain about how to identify T-units, we recommend that you first complete the training exercises in Section III. There is no digital audio file for responses to this subtest because the students produce written responses on the *Student Response Form*. In this section, practice examples are provided for Student 1 (age 6;9) for Story A, Student 3 (age 9) for Story B, Student 4 (age 12) for Story C, and Student 5 (age 14) for Story D; you will need a blank *Examiner Record Form,* but for your convenience, there is a blank content units scoring form included for each story example. Additional examples of how to score WE stories are included in Section III.

After completing the training exercises in Section III, score the practice samples for Stories A–D. This will require several steps.

- *Step 1:* Identify the content units included in the rewritten story by circling 1 for each content unit the student included.

- *Step 2:* Divide this by the number of possible content units and multiply by 100 to calculate the percentage of content units included. This is the Written Expression–Discourse score (WE-Disc).

- *Step 3:* Identify the T-units by placing a slash after each T-unit or fragment.

- *Step 4:* Divide the number of content units by the number of T-units (and round the number to 2 decimals) to calculate the number of content units per T-unit. This is the Written Expression–Sentence score (WE-Sent).

- *Step 5:* Identify and circle any error words, which include misspelled words, words with backward letters, words with punctuation errors, words that do not fit the grammatical context, and words that are omitted but are needed to make a sentence grammatical.

- *Step 6:* Count the total words produced by the student in the body of the story.

WE

WRITTEN EXPRESSION

- *Step 7:* Calculate the percentage of words produced without error by subtracting the error words from total words, dividing this number by total words, and multiplying the quotient by 100. This is the Written Expression–Word score (WE-Word).

Ask yourself the following questions as you complete the exercise:

1. Under what circumstances should I read the facts of the student's story aloud to him or her immediately before the student is asked to begin rewriting the facts to sound less choppy and more interesting? What must I have students do immediately prior to administering the subtest?

2. When counting content units to calculate the Written Expression–Discourse score (WE-Disc), can a student get credit for a content unit if he or she uses *one* of the underlined words shown in the content unit scoring table but not *all* of them? Can the student get credit for using synonyms on this subtest?

3. What should I do if the student declines to do the task or writes only a single word or sentence and then says he or she is done? What should I do if the student takes an excessively long time to complete this task (i.e., more than 20 minutes)?

4. When marking T-units, what should I do with fragments (i.e., grammatical units that are less than a main clause)? Should I put a slash mark wherever the student puts end punctuation, such as a period, question mark, or exclamation point?

5. When marking error words, what should I do if the student orients a letter in the wrong direction? What should I do if the student makes an error of capitalization? What if the student spells a word correctly but adds a plural, possessive, or verb ending that does not fit the grammatical context or omits one of these inflectional morphemes? What should I do if the student writes a title and misspells one of the words in the title?

6. When counting total words, should I count any words in the title or an ending, such as "the end"?

7. Based on the comparison of my results to the scoring examples, which content units, T-units, or error words decisions do I find most challenging to score?

The class pet it was a hamster. The hamster has spots the spots are brown and white it got out it was last week the door and the cage was open. they found him thay put him back in his cage. They closed the door he went to sleep.

<table>
<tr><td colspan="6" align="center">WRITTEN EXPRESSION CONTENT UNITS SCORING FORM
Story A: "The Class Pet" (p. 69)</td></tr>
<tr><td>1. The <u>class</u> has a <u>pet</u>.</td><td>0</td><td>1</td><td>9. The <u>door</u> was open.</td><td>0</td><td>1</td></tr>
<tr><td>2. It is a <u>hamster</u>.</td><td>0</td><td>1</td><td>10. The children <u>looked</u>.</td><td>0</td><td>1</td></tr>
<tr><td>3. The hamster has <u>spots</u>.</td><td>0</td><td>1</td><td>11. The children <u>found</u> him.</td><td>0</td><td>1</td></tr>
<tr><td>4. Some are <u>brown</u>.</td><td>0</td><td>1</td><td>12. They <u>put him back</u>.</td><td>0</td><td>1</td></tr>
<tr><td>5. Some are <u>white</u>.</td><td>0</td><td>1</td><td>13. They put him in the <u>cage</u>.</td><td>0</td><td>1</td></tr>
<tr><td>6. It <u>got out</u>.</td><td>0</td><td>1</td><td>14. They closed the <u>door</u>.</td><td>0</td><td>1</td></tr>
<tr><td>7. It was one day <u>last week</u>.</td><td>0</td><td>1</td><td>15. He found a <u>corner</u>.</td><td>0</td><td>1</td></tr>
<tr><td>8. The cage was <u>open</u>.</td><td>0</td><td>1</td><td>16. He went to <u>sleep</u>.</td><td>0</td><td>1</td></tr>
<tr><td></td><td></td><td></td><td align="right">Content Units total</td><td></td><td>/16</td></tr>
</table>

6;6–7

Discourse Score	_____ Content Units / 16 possible × 100 = _____% Content Included
Sentence Score	_____ Content Units / _____ T-units* = _____ Sentence Score (record 2 decimal places)
Word Score	_____ Total Words − _____ Error Words = _____ Total Correct Words / _____ Total Words × 100 = _____% Words Correct

Note: For more information about how to calculate T-units, see pages 74–77 in the *Examiner's Manual.*
Qualitative observations:

Note: Examiner reread the story to student because not all words were read correctly by the student on Subtest 11, Reading Fluency

Written Expression (WE) Story A response produced by Student 1,
a 6-year, 9-month-old boy and blank scoring form for practice exercise.

treat as 1 T-unit

The class pet | it was a hamster | the hamster
has spots | the spots are brown and white | it got out |
it was last week | the door and the cage was open |
they found him | they put him back in his cage |
They closed the door | he went to sleep |

6;6–7

WRITTEN EXPRESSION CONTENT UNITS SCORING FORM					
Story A: "The Class Pet" (p. 69)					
1. The class has a pet.	0	(1)	9. The door was open.	0	(1)
2. It is a hamster.	0	(1)	10. The children looked.	(0)	1
3. The hamster has spots.	0	(1)	11. The children found him.	0	(1)
4. Some are brown.	0	(1)	12. They put him back.	0	(1)
5. Some are white.	0	(1)	13. They put him in the cage.	0	(1)
6. It got out.	0	(1)	14. They closed the door.	0	(1)
7. It was one day last week.	0	(1)	15. He found a corner.	(0)	1
8. The cage was open.	0	(1)	16. He went to sleep.	0	(1)
				Content Units total	14 /16

Discourse Score	14 Content Units / 16 possible × 100 = 88 % Content Included
Sentence Score	14 Content Units / 9 T-units* = 1.56 Sentence Score (record 2 decimal places)
Word Score	49 Total Words − 2 Error Words = 47 Total Correct Words / 49 Total Words × 100 = 96 % Words Correct

*Note: For more information about how to calculate T-units, see pages 74–77 in the *Examiner's Manual*.

Qualitative observations:
Note: Examiner reread the story to student because not all words were read correctly by the student on Subtest II, Reading Fluency

Written Expression (WE) Story A scored for Student 1, a 6-year, 9-month-boy with normal language.

We have a. Pranceble The Prancelble has a dater. her name is Sara. She whantid to be a Clown. she Came on monday. she came to our scoole. She had makeup. She had a wig. A ball was on her nowse. I thas red. it was big. She looked scary. She wallkt in to a class The chigrin were ehong. The chilgrin saw her. some chilgrin cride They were scard. She took of her wig. The chilgrih were happy. They know sara.

WRITTEN EXPRESSION CONTENT UNITS SCORING FORM						
Story B: "The Principal's Daughter" (p. 71)						
1. We have a principal.	0	1	11. It was big.	0	1	
2. The principal has a daughter.	0	1	12. She looked scary.	0	1	
3. Her name is Sara.	0	1	13. She walked into a class.	0	1	
4. She wants to be a clown.	0	1	14. The children were young.	0	1	
5. She came Monday.	0	1	15. The children saw her.	0	1	
6. She came to our school.	0	1	16. Some children cried.	0	1	
7. She had on makeup.	0	1	17. They were scared.	0	1	
8. She had on a wig.*	0	1	18. She took off her wig.	0	1	
9. A ball was on her nose.	0	1	19. The children were happy.	0	1	
10. It was red.	0	1	20. They knew Sara.	0	1	
				Content Units total	/20	

*Note: If child writes "dress" or "attire," score 1 for wig but 0 for makeup or ball on nose.

Discourse Score	____ Content Units / 20 possible × 100 = ____% Content Included
Sentence Score	____ Content Units / ____ T-units* = ____ Sentence Score (record 2 decimal places)
Word Score	____ Total Words − ____ Error Words = ____ Total Correct Words / ____ Total Words × 100 = ____% Words Correct

*Note: For more information about how to calculate T-units, see pages 74–77 in the *Examiner's Manual*.

Qualitative observations:

I tried to point out the difference in practice story vs example.
She was very systematic about copying.
But misspelled many words.
Commented that the subtest was fun!

Written Expression (WE) Story B response produced by Student 3,
a 9-year-old girl and blank scoring form for practice exercise.

WE

WRITTEN EXPRESSION

We have a.
(Pranceble) The (Prancelble) has a (dater)
her name is Sara. She (whantid) to be
a clown. she Came on monday.
she came to our (scoole.) she had makeup.
she had a wig. A ball was on her (nowse)
I thas red. it was big. She looked scary.
she (wallkt) in to a class The (chigrin) were
young
(hong) The (chilgrin) saw her, some (chilgrin) (cride.)
They were (scard.) she took (of) her wig.
The (chitgrih) were happy, They (know) sara.

8–10	WRITTEN EXPRESSION CONTENT UNITS SCORING FORM					
	Story B: "The Principal's Daughter" (p. 71)					
	1. We have a principal.	0	(1)	11. It was big.	0	(1)
	2. The principal has a daughter.	0	(1)	12. She looked scary.	0	(1)
	3. Her name is Sara.	0	(1)	13. She walked into a class.	0	(1)
	4. She wants to be a clown.	0	(1)	14. The children were young.	0	(1)
	5. She came Monday.	0	(1)	15. The children saw her.	0	(1)
	6. She came to our school.	0	(1)	16. Some children cried.	0	(1)
	7. She had on makeup.	0	(1)	17. They were scared.	0	(1)
	8. She had on a wig.*	0	(1)	18. She took off her wig.	0	(1)
	9. A ball was on her nose.	0	(1)	19. The children were happy.	0	(1)
	10. It was red.	0	(1)	20. They knew Sara.	0	(1)
				Content Units total		20 /20

*Note: If child writes "dress" or "attire," score 1 for wig but 0 for makeup or ball on nose.

Discourse Score	20 Content Units / 20 possible × 100 = 100% Content Included
Sentence Score	20 Content Units / 20 T-units* = 1.0 Sentence Score (record 2 decimal places)
Word Score	81 Total Words − 16 Error Words = 65 Total Correct Words / 81 Total Words × 100 = 80 % Words Correct

*Note: For more information about how to calculate T-units, see pages 74–77 in the Examiner's Manual.

Qualitative observations:

I tried to point out the difference in practice story vs example.
She was very systematic about copying.
But misspelled many words.
Commented that the subtest was fun!

Written Expression (WE) Story B scored for Student 3,
a 9-year-old girl with language learning disability.

> Our school, was closed last Wednesday. It was a school day but it was closed all day. The Janitor came in at 6 A.M, but when he opened the doors he smelled something so strong it almost knocked him over. It. Was. A. Skunk. Duhn duhn duh! He left the doors open while he searched the library + cafeteria. In the cafeteria he found to of them, who had eaten so many cookies, they looked full. He immediatley called animal control. The animal control workers came right away, captured the skunks, and released them in the woods. The smell stayed in the building for 1 week. Then the school finally smelled normal.

11–13

WRITTEN EXPRESSION CONTENT UNITS SCORING FORM					
Story C: "When the School Closed" (p. 73)					
1. Our <u>school</u> was <u>closed</u>.	0	1	17. There were <u>two</u>.	0	1
2. It was last <u>Wednesday</u>.	0	1	18. They were eating <u>cookies</u>.	0	1
3. It was a <u>school day</u>.	0	1	19. They had <u>eaten many</u>.	0	1
4. It was <u>closed all day</u>.	0	1	20. They looked <u>full</u>.	0	1
5. The <u>janitor came in</u> at <u>6</u> <u>a.m.</u>	0	1	21. He called <u>animal control</u>.	0	1
6. He <u>opened</u> the <u>school</u>.	0	1	22. He called <u>right away</u>.	0	1
7. He <u>smelled</u> something.	0	1	23. The <u>workers</u> came.	0	1
8. It was <u>strong</u>.	0	1	24. They <u>took</u> the <u>skunks</u>.	0	1
9. It almost <u>knocked him over</u>. (figurative meaning)	0	1	25. They <u>let</u> them <u>go</u>.	0	1
10. It was a <u>skunk</u>.	0	1	26. It was in the <u>woods</u>.	0	1
11. He <u>opened</u> the <u>doors</u>.	0	1	27. The <u>smell stayed</u>.	0	1
12. He <u>left them</u> open.	0	1	28. It was in the <u>building</u>.	0	1
13. He <u>searched</u>. (looked in)	0	1	29. The smell <u>finally left</u>.	0	1
14. He looked in the <u>library</u>.	0	1	30. It took <u>one week</u>.	0	1
15. He looked in the <u>cafeteria</u>.	0	1	31. The <u>school</u> smelled <u>normal</u>.	0	1
16. He <u>found</u> the <u>skunks</u>.	0	1	**Content Units total**		**/31**

Discourse Score	____ Content Units / 31 possible × 100 = ____% Content Included
Sentence Score	____ Content Units / ____ T-units* = ____ Sentence Score (record 2 decimal places)
Word Score	____ Total Words – ____ Error Words = ____ Total Correct Words / ____ Total Words × 100 = ____% Words Correct

Note: For more information about how to calculate T-units, see pages 74–77 in the *Examiner's Manual.*
Qualitative observations:

Written Expression (WE) Story C response produced by Student 4,
a 12-year-old boy and blank scoring form for practice exercise.

Our school, was closed last Wednesday. / It was a school day / but it was closed all day. / The janitor came in at 6 A.M. / but when he opened the doors he smelled something so strong it almost knocked him over. / It. Was. A. Skunk. Duhn duhn duh! / He left the doors open while he searched the library + cafeteria. / In the cafeteria he found (to) of them, who had eaten so many cookies, they looked full. / He (immediatley) called animal control. / The animal control workers came right away, captured the skunks, and released them in the woods. / The smell stayed in the building for 1 week. / Then the school finally smelled normal. /

WRITTEN EXPRESSION CONTENT UNITS SCORING FORM
Story C: "When the School Closed" (p. 73)

11–13

	0	1		0	1
1. Our school was closed.	0	(1)	17. There were two.	0	(1)
2. It was last Wednesday.	0	(1)	18. They were eating cookies.	0	(1)
3. It was a school day.	0	(1)	19. They had eaten many.	0	(1)
4. It was closed all day.	0	(1)	20. They looked full.	0	(1)
5. The janitor came in at 6 a.m.	0	(1)	21. He called animal control.	0	(1)
6. He opened the school.	0	(1)	22. He called right away.	0	(1)
7. He smelled something.	0	(1)	23. The workers came.	0	(1)
8. It was strong.	0	(1)	24. They took the skunks.	0	(1)
9. It almost knocked him over. (figurative meaning)	0	(1)	25. They let them go.	0	(1)
10. It was a skunk.	0	(1)	26. It was in the woods.	0	(1)
11. He opened the doors.	0	(1)	27. The smell stayed.	0	(1)
12. He left them open.	0	(1)	28. It was in the building.	0	(1)
13. He searched. (looked in)	0	(1)	29. The smell finally left.	0	(1)
14. He looked in the library.	0	(1)	30. It took one week.	0	(1)
15. He looked in the cafeteria.	0	(1)	31. The school smelled normal.	0	(1)
16. He found the skunks.	0	(1)	**Content Units total**	**31**	**/31**

Discourse Score	__31__ Content Units / 31 possible × 100 = __100__% Content Included
Sentence Score	__31__ Content Units / __12__ T-units* = __2.58__ Sentence Score (record 2 decimal places)
Word Score	__110__ Total Words − __2__ Error Words = __108__ Total Correct Words / __110__ Total Words × 100 = __98__% Words Correct

Note: For more information about how to calculate T-units, see pages 74–77 in the *Examiner's Manual*.
Qualitative observations:
"duhn-duhn-duh" counted as one word.
"It. Was. A. Skunk." counted as one t-unit.

**Written Expression (WE) Story C scored for
Student 4, a 12-year-old boy with normal language.**

The Building

There was an old building, no one knew exactly how old it was, because they had no records. But people talked about it, because it had a history. Some people knew it was used long ago, in a war In that war it ~~served~~ surved as an hospital. Hundreds of soldiers came there, many were treated, but many died. Those who died were burried behind the building, It is still there today. People did'nt care or think about it. It was almost hidden. Then something happened that made them change their opinions The city needed a new road, so they were going to demolish the building so they could have the land. But now that the people cared they did everything they could to stop it. They wrote articles gave speaches, raised money, saved the building and the graveyard. But that wasnt the only thing they saved, they also saved something more important, their history.

WRITTEN EXPRESSION CONTENT UNITS SCORING FORM

Story D: "The Building" (p. 75)

14+

1. There was a <u>building</u>.	0	1	18. People <u>did not think</u> about it.	0	1
2. It was <u>old</u>.	0	1	19. It was almost <u>hidden</u>.	0	1
3. <u>No one knew</u> how old.	0	1	20. They did <u>not care</u>.	0	1
4. There were <u>no records</u>.	0	1	21. Then <u>something happened</u>.	0	1
5. <u>People talked</u> about it.	0	1	22. The <u>city wanted</u> the <u>land</u>.	0	1
6. It had a <u>history</u>.	0	1	23. They needed a <u>new road</u>.	0	1
7. <u>Some</u> people <u>knew</u>.	0	1	24. The <u>building</u> would be <u>demolished</u>.	0	1
8. It was used in a <u>war</u>.	0	1	25. People suddenly <u>cared</u>.	0	1
9. It was <u>long ago</u>.	0	1	26. They wrote <u>articles</u>.	0	1
10. The building was a <u>hospital</u>.	0	1	27. They gave <u>speeches</u>.	0	1
11. <u>Soldiers came</u> there.	0	1	28. They raised <u>money</u>.	0	1
12. There were <u>hundreds</u>.	0	1	29. They <u>saved</u> the <u>building</u>.	0	1
13. Many were <u>treated</u>.	0	1	30. They saved the <u>graveyard</u>.*	0	1
14. Many <u>died</u>.	0	1	31. They saved <u>something else</u>.	0	1
15. They were <u>buried</u>.	0	1	32. It was their <u>history</u>.	0	1
16. The <u>graveyard</u> was <u>still</u> there.*	0	1	33. That was more <u>important</u>.	0	1
17. It was <u>behind</u> the <u>building</u>.	0	1	**Content Units total**		/33

Note: Count graveyard as one word when counting total words for Written Expression regardless of spacing.

Discourse Score	____ Content Units / 33 possible × 100 = ____% Content Included
Sentence Score	____ Content Units / ____ T-units* = ____ Sentence Score (record 2 decimal places)
Word Score	____ Total Words − ____ Error Words = ____ Total Correct Words / ____ Total Words × 100 = ____ % Words Correct

Note: For more information about how to calculate T-units, see pages 74–77 in the *Examiner's Manual.*

Qualitative observations:

WRITTEN EXPRESSION

Written Expression (WE) Story D response produced by Student 5,
a 14-year-old girl and blank scoring form for practice exercise.

The Building

There was an old building, no one knew exactly how old it was, because they had no records. But people talked about it, because it had a history. Some people knew it was used long ago in a war. In that war it ~~surved~~ as ~~an~~ hospital. Hundreds of ~~soldiers~~ came there, many were treated, but many died. Those who died were ~~burried~~ behind the building. It is still there today. People didn't care or think about it. It was almost hidden. Then something happened that made them change their opinions. The city needed a new road, so they were going to demolish the building so they could have the land. But the people cared they did everything they could to stop it. They wrote articles gave ~~speaches~~, raised money, saved the building and the graveyard. But that wasn't the only thing they saved, they also saved something more important, their history.

WRITTEN EXPRESSION CONTENT UNITS SCORING FORM					
Story D: "The Building" (p. 75)					
1. There was a <u>building</u>.	0	(1)	18. People <u>did not think</u> about it.	0	(1)
2. It was <u>old</u>.	0	(1)	19. It was almost <u>hidden</u>.	0	(1)
3. <u>No one knew</u> how old.	0	(1)	20. They did <u>not care</u>.	0	(1)
4. There were <u>no records</u>.	0	(1)	21. Then <u>something happened</u>.	0	(1)
5. <u>People talked</u> about it.	0	(1)	22. The <u>city wanted</u> the <u>land</u>.	0	(1)
6. It had a <u>history</u>.	0	(1)	23. They needed a <u>new road</u>.	0	(1)
7. <u>Some</u> people <u>knew</u>.	0	(1)	24. The <u>building</u> would be <u>demolished</u>.	0	(1)
8. It was used in a <u>war</u>.	0	(1)	25. People suddenly <u>cared</u>.	0	(1)
9. It was <u>long ago</u>.	0	(1)	26. They wrote <u>articles</u>.	0	(1)
10. The building was a <u>hospital</u>.	0	(1)	27. They gave <u>speeches</u>.	0	(1)
11. <u>Soldiers came</u> there.	0	(1)	28. They raised <u>money</u>.	0	(1)
12. There were <u>hundreds</u>.	0	(1)	29. They <u>saved</u> the <u>building</u>.	0	(1)
13. Many were <u>treated</u>.	0	(1)	30. They saved the <u>graveyard</u>.*	0	(1)
14. Many <u>died</u>.	0	(1)	31. They saved <u>something else</u>.	0	(1)
15. They were <u>buried</u>.	0	(1)	32. It was their <u>history</u>.	0	(1)
16. The <u>graveyard</u> was <u>still</u> there.*	0	(1)	33. That was more <u>important</u>.	0	(1)
17. It was <u>behind</u> the <u>building</u>.	0	(1)	**Content Units total**		33 /33

*Note: Count graveyard as one word when counting total words for Written Expression regardless of spacing.

Discourse Score	33 Content Units / 33 possible × 100 = 100 % Content Included
Sentence Score	33 Content Units / 19 T-units* = 1.74 Sentence Score (record 2 decimal places)
Word Score	154 Total Words − 5 Error Words = 149 Total Correct Words / 154 Total Words × 100 = 97 % Words Correct

*Note: For more information about how to calculate T-units, see pages 74–77 in the Examiner's Manual.

Qualitative observations:

Written Expression (WE) Story D scored for Student 5, a 14-year-old girl with normal language.

ANSWERS

Make your best effort to complete the exercise before you read the following answers:

1. Read aloud the facts of the student's story immediately prior to asking the student to begin writing only if the student misreads or cannot decode any of the words for the Reading Fluency (RF) subtest. The examiner rereads all the facts of the story for Student 1 because the student had difficulty reading the words "cage" (even though it was self-corrected) and "corner," which was not decoded. All students must complete the RF subtest immediately prior to beginning the WE subtest. If the student cannot read any of the words on the RF subtest, reread the full set of facts to the student immediately before asking him or her to begin rewriting the story.

2. When counting content units, you may decide to award a student credit for the content unit even if he or she does not use all of the underlined words. This decision is appropriate when you judge that the student has represented the meaning captured in that content unit but worded it slightly differently. This includes giving credit for synonyms or a different way of expressing the same content. An example would be to give credit for "He opened the doors" and "He left them open" if a student writes "He left the doors open all day."

3. If a student declines to do the task or writes only a single word or sentence, do whatever you can to encourage the student to attempt the task. If the student puts his or her pencil down, indicates that he or she is finished, and declines to proceed despite encouragement, stop and score any material produced. If the student declines to attempt the task despite encouragement, enter the Discourse, Sentence, and Word raw scores as 0 and compare them to normative data. This can provide baseline data for when you readminister the TILLS to the student 6 months or more in the future, hopefully following intervention. If a student takes more than 20 minutes to complete this task, you should say, "I'd like you to finish the sentence you're on and then we can be done with this one." If the student still insists on completing the story, allow the student to continue, and score the entire attempt.

4. When marking T-units, fragments can be challenging. It is important to avoid either inflating the T-unit count by marking fragments as separate units or deflating the T-unit count by treating them as part of other units. It is best to treat one- or two-word fragments as part of adjacent T-units but to count longer phrases as stand-alone, incomplete T-units (also called C-units). Another tip for marking T-units is to score the samples as if they were produced orally rather than considering the student's end punctuation.

5. When marking error words, you should circle any word with a letter oriented in the wrong direction and count it as an error word. This applies not only to letters that change identity with orientation, such as *b-d* and *p-q* confusions, but also misorientation of letters such as *s* or *c,* which do not result in a different letter. If you think this rule might be inflating a student's error score, make note to that effect under Qualitative Observations; however, you must score the subtest in the way it was standardized to be able to compare the student's score to the norms. A consistent problem of this nature might point to an area that should be targeted in intervention. Errors of capitalization do not affect scoring. Circle any word that is inflected incorrectly for the sentence context (i.e., with omitted or extraneous plural, possessive, or verb tense markers). Do not circle any word the student misspells in a segment that is clearly meant to be a title or "the end."

6. Do not count words in titles or closure statements, such as "the end," in total word counts or in T-unit counts.

7. The following are some of the challenging issues and important points that you should apply when scoring this exercise for students of different ages.

Story A Scoring

- *Story A, content units:* Content unit scoring is fairly straightforward for Student 1, a 6-year, 9-month-old boy with normal language. He includes all of the original content units except for indicating that the children "looked" and the hamster found a "corner." This yields a Written Expression–Discourse score (WE-Disc) of 88%.

- *Story A, T-units:* Nine T-units are marked and counted. The first T-unit is "The class pet it was a hamster." Scoring this one is a bit challenging because the first three words repeat the title. However, the student does not format this as a title, so it is not treated as such. In this grammatical construction, the words "the class pet" function as a dependent phrase attached to the main clause, "it was a hamster," describing the referent for the pronoun, "it." The student combines a few content units into more complex T-units, mostly by forming compound adjective phrases (e.g., "the spots are brown and white") and compound noun phrases (e.g., "the door and the cage was open"). The student's Written Expression–Sentence score (WE-Sent) of 1.56 reflects his ability to combine the 14 rewritten content units into a smaller number of 9 T-units.

- *Story A, error words:* Although the sentence with the compound noun phrase "the door and the cage was open" is awkward, it is credited for content units without penalty (following the rule of giving credit when in doubt); however, a word error is marked for "was," which should have been "were" due to the compound subject. Therefore, this student produces only two error words, *was/were* (which also would have been identified as an error word due to the backward *s*) and *thay/they*.

- *Story A, total words:* The total word count (49 words) is fairly straightforward for this story. The count of correct words is 47, and the Written Expression–Word score (WE-Word) is 47/49 = 96%, which is high for a 6-year-old. The WE-Word score may be influenced by a particularly low total word count. If a student produces few words but makes no errors, the WE-Word score of 100% might seem inflated for the student's ability. If the student produces only a few words but makes errors on half of them, the WE-Word score of 50% might appear to be lower than warranted. When normative data are used to standardize these scores, however, they may seem more reasonable. In any case, you may describe qualitative aspects of a student's performance to augment information from the student's quantitative scores. The advantages of a norm-referenced test depend on scoring the test as it was standardized.

Story B Scoring

- *Story B, content units:* Student 3, a 9-year-old girl with language learning disability, includes all of the original content units in the rewritten story, but she does so by copying them. When this occurs, you may look for evidence that the student actually understood what she was writing. You can infer this if the student makes minor changes in the text that maintain the original meaning. When a student copies with few changes, however, it is difficult to know to what degree the student has comprehended the story and could reformulate it without copying. In this example, the student makes word-level changes but otherwise keeps the original sentence structure. Still, she demonstrates strength in staying with the task. She also comments that it "was fun," suggesting a possible modality for working on language and spelling skills in intervention. Further probing of written language following TILLS testing could provide additional valuable information about the student's written language ability.

- *Story B, T-units:* Counting T-units is straightforward when a student copies the original T-units. Exact or nearly exact copying yields a Written Expression–Sentence score (WE-Sent) of 1.0. In this example, the student essentially copies all 20 of the 20 original T-units for a WE-Sent score of 20/20 = 1.0. The examiner makes a note about how she tried to handle this, "I tried to point out the differences between the facts in the practice story and the example." The examiner adds that in spite of this, "she was very systematic about copying." If you notice that a student is simply copying when you are administering this subtest, try reminding the student about the nature of the task, but then let him or her proceed independently.

- *Story B, error words:* The student makes a number of word errors of different types, despite the fact that the *Stimulus Book* remains open so that the facts of the story (with models of correctly spelled words) are visible to the student. Misspellings include the following: *pranceble/principal, prancelble/principal, dater/daughter, whantid/wanted, scoole/school, nose/nowse, walkt/walked, chigrin/children, ehong/young, chilgrin/children* (three times), *cride/cried, scard/scared, of/off,* and *know/knew.* Listing words in this manner, with the misspelling compared to the target, can help you identify patterns of difficulty that you could investigate further in informal curriculum-based assessment following the TILLS. In this case, among other problems, the student consistently misspells the *-ed* verb tense ending, which should be examined further in informal follow-up assessment.

- *Story B, total words:* Because this student writes 81 total words and misspells 16 of them, the student's WE-Word score was 81 − 16 = 54/81 = 80% words written correctly.

Story C Scoring

- *Story C, content units:* Student 4, a 12-year-old boy with normal language, incorporates all of the original content units, as the prior student in the Story B example does. In this case, however, the student does so without copying. This makes some scoring decisions a bit more complex. For example, the original facts for Items 6–9 read as follows: "He opened the school," "He smelled something," "It was strong," and "It almost knocked him over." The student incorporates the essential meaning for all four of these content units in the combined T-unit, "But when he opened the doors he smelled something so strong it almost knocked him over." As the underlined words show, almost all of the key words are present in the revised sentence. The exception is that the student wrote "he opened the *doors*" rather than "he opened the *school*." Because the student captures the essential meaning with these revised words, he is was given credit for Content Unit 6. A similar scoring decision is made to give credit for Content Units 27–31: "The smell stayed," "It was in the building," "The smell finally left," "It took one week," "The school smelled normal." This decision is based on the student's 2 T-unit combination, "The smell stayed in the building for 1 week. Then the school finally smelled normal."

- *Story C, T-units:* This student does something interesting with end punctuation for dramatic effect. He writes, "It. Was. A. Skunk." followed by the sound effect "Duhn Duhn Duh." This element of originality is delightful, but it presents a scoring challenge to the examiner. It is a good example of when one should ignore the student's punctuation. The examiner decided to incorporate the sound effect (Duhn Duhn Duh) into the T-unit it accompanied, thus treating this entire construction as a single T-unit. The rationale for this decision was to avoid inflating the T-unit count by counting the sound effect as a separate fragment. That would have the effect of increasing the denominator and deflating the Written Expression–Sentence score (WE-Sent).

- *Story C, error words:* The student makes two spelling errors, spelling *to/two* and *immediatley/immediately.*

- *Story C, total words:* Numerals are counted as single words in the total word count. This student produces 110 total words – 2 error words = 108/110, for 98% words correct.

Story D Scoring

- *Story D, content units:* Student 5, a 14-year-old girl with normal language, incorporates all 33 of the original content units into the rewritten story.

- *Story D, T-units:* The student demonstrates that she understands the task and shows effective sentence-combining skills by rewriting the original 33 T-units into fewer (19), but more complex, T-units. This yields a WE-Sent score of 33/19 = 1.74. The student's example illustrates the difference between using coordinating conjunctions, such as *but* and *so,* to coordinate separate T-units and using a subordinating conjunction, such as *because,* to add a dependent clause to an independent clause within the same T-unit. Consider the T-unit "So they were going to demolish the building so they could have the land." This illustrates both the coordinating use of the conjunction *so* at the beginning of the sentence and the subordinating use of *so* with the meaning "so that" to introduce a clause that is dependent to the main clause "they were going to demolish the building."

- *Story D, error words:* Five error words are identified and circled. One of them is a usage error, in which the student writes "an hospital" rather than "a hospital."

- *Story D, total words:* The total word count is 154. The WE-Word score is calculated as follows: 154 total words – 5 error words = 149 total correct words/154 total words = 97%.

For further scored examples for this subtest, see Section III.

WE

WRITTEN EXPRESSION

RECAP OF SUBTEST

The Social Communication (SC) subtest requires the student to be an actor. He or she listens to the examiner read a short "scene" while viewing the same words in the *Stimulus Book*. The student then says what one of the characters in the scene would say and says it how the character would say it. An example is used to demonstrate acting out a child whining when the child's mother will not let him or her buy candy in the grocery store.

Use as a stand-alone measure: Yes	**Start rule:** Start points for age ranges are indicated by arrows.
Average time to administer: 9 minutes	**Basal rule:** 6 consecutive scores of 1
Materials: *Examiner Record Form* (pp. 32–35), *Stimulus Book* (pp. 80–107 for boys; pp. 108–135 for girls), audio recording device (recommended)	**Ceiling rule:** 6 scores of 0 out of 8 consecutive items
	Repetition: Allowed
	Probes: Yes (as specified in the *Examiner's Manual*)

PRACTICE EXERCISE

To complete this exercise, you will need Track 12 from the Examiner's Practice Workbook Audio Files folder on the *Digital Audio Files* (USB drive) for Student 1, a 6-year, 9-month-old boy with normal language. Listen to the test administration on the audio file and score Student 1's responses using a blank *Examiner Record Form*.

Ask yourself the following questions as you complete the exercise:

1. What score does a student earn if he or she gets only the vocabulary or the pragmatic element of a scene correct but not both? For example, what should the item score be if the student earns credit for only the vocabulary aspect but uses the wrong tone of voice? What should the score be if the student gets the expected tone of voice but changes the meaning?

2. The start point for Student 1 is Item 1. What is the start point for a 16-year-old? What if the 16-year-old gets Item 6 correct but then makes an error on Item 7? What should I do next?

3. Why is it a mistake for the examiner to say, "Good arguing" to the student after Item 2?

4. Why does the examiner decline to define *criticize* for the student on Item 8 when the student indicates that he does not know the meaning of the word?

5. What is the ceiling rule? Does the examiner discontinue testing exactly at the ceiling? If not, why? What would the examiner need to do if the student had gotten an item correct after reaching the ceiling?

6. Which items do I find challenging to score? What is my rationale for my scoring decisions?

ANSWERS

Make your best effort to complete the exercise before you read the following answers:

1. To earn an item score of 1, the student must meet scoring criteria both for vocabulary *and* pragmatics in formulating a response to the item. That is, the student

must represent both the linguistic (vocabulary and semantics) and paralinguistic (pragmatic aspects of tone of voice, directiveness, etc.) aspects of social communication specified in the presented scenario. If the student earns 0 on either subcomponent, the item score is 0. The item score can be 1 only if the student earns a score of 1 for both vocabulary and pragmatics.

2. You should start with Item 6 if you are testing a 16-year-old. If the 16-year-old gets Item 6 correct but then makes an error on Item 7, you should flip back to Item 5 and then continue testing previous items until you administer Item 1. The basal rule is six items consecutively correct, which cannot occur for this student until Item 1. After administering Item 1, consider the basal met, whether or not the student made any errors on Items 1–5. Then, return to Item 8 and test it and consecutive items until you establish a ceiling or have administered all 13 items.

3. There are two reasons why it was a bad idea for the examiner to say, "Good arguing," to the student after Item 2. The first is that, throughout testing, examiners should give only general encouragement, such as "you're doing a nice job" or "you've got the idea," rather than saying something specific about the nature of the performance. The second is that the student seemed to respond to this praise by continuing to use that particular voice on subsequent items. The examiner tried to repair this mistake by reminding the student not to use the same voice for all the different scenes, which was an acceptable way of handling this.

4. Examiners are not allowed to define terms for students on any TILLS subtest, either during or after testing. Part of the Social Communication (SC) subtest score depends on knowing the vocabulary for describing different communicative intentions, as well as how to represent those intentions with language and tone of voice.

5. The ceiling rule is to cease testing only if a student earns an item score of 0 on six out of eight consecutive items. In this case, the examiner continues testing one item beyond the ceiling because she is uncertain in the moment how to score the student's response to Item 12. Therefore, the examiner administers Item 13 to be sure to establish a ceiling. If the student had earned a score of 1 on Item 13, the examiner would have had to treat it as 0 because it occurred after the ceiling.

6. Interesting and challenging items include the following:

   • *Item 1:* Score 1 because the student represents the intended meaning about both bragging and the dog's size and uses a bragging tone of voice. The rule of thumb is not to be too picky about dramatization of the tone of voice because some students are shy and not willing to extend themselves to be highly dramatic.

   • *Item 2:* Score 1 because brief responses are acceptable if they capture the essence of the vocabulary and pragmatics.

   • *Item 3:* Score 1 because a student can earn credit for disagreeing with any aspect of the friend's plan, as this student does.

   • *Item 4:* Score 1 because the student must specify a punishment but does not have to comment on the noise to earn credit on this item.

   • *Item 5:* Score 0 because politely turning down an invitation requires indirectness and a plausible excuse.

   • *Item 6:* Score 1. This item is challenging. To earn credit, the student must demand to be the goalie, but demanding can be conveyed by tone of voice, as the examiner judges this student to do when he says, "I wanna be the goalie."

- *Item 7:* Score 0 because although the student uses an ordering tone of voice, adding "please" at the end softens the order, making it into a request.

- *Item 8:* Score 0 because the student expresses that he does not know the meaning of the key vocabulary term *criticize*.

- *Item 9:* Score 0 because the student comments that this is a "hard one," so the examiner moves on after pausing to allow him to give it a try, which he does not elect to do.

- *Item 10:* Score 0 because the student takes the role of the talk show host but then comments on himself rather than saying something flattering about the guest.

- *Item 11:* Score 1. This item can be challenging to score. Even if the verbal message is all about what the friend should do differently in the future, as long as it is said in an encouraging tone, the student earns credit for the item.

- *Item 12:* Score 0. The examiner was not sure at first how to score "Aren't you going to give me a compliment?" Upon reflection, it was clear that, although this was fishing, it was too direct. It would be socially unusual to ask directly for a compliment, whereas asking, "How do you like my new clothes?" or even "Aren't you going to say something about my new clothes?" would be fishing for a compliment.

- *Item 13:* Score 0 because although the student claims some knowledge of the term *sarcastic,* he is not able to act it out. Because this item is past the ceiling, it would be scored 0 even if he is able to do it, which would be rare for a 6-year-old.

6–11

1. *(for girls)* Sally's friend always <u>brags</u> about her dog. One day Sally decides to top her friend's bragging by telling how big her own dog is. What do you think Sally would say?

1. *(for boys)* Sam's friend always <u>brags</u> about his dog. One day Sam decides to top his friend's bragging by telling how big his own dog is. What do you think Sam would say?

Student's response:	Vocabulary	Pragmatics	Item Score	
Brags about dog's size in a bragging tone.	(1)	(1)		
My dog's a lot bigger than yours.	0	0	0	(1)

2. *(for girls)* Rita wants to <u>argue</u> with her friend about whose turn it is to go first playing a game. What do you think Rita would say?

2. *(for boys)* Rick wants to <u>argue</u> with his friend about whose turn it is to go first playing a game. What do you think Rick would say?

Student's response:	Vocabulary	Pragmatics	Item Score	
Insists on taking a turn in an argumentative tone.	(1)	(1)		
I wanna go first.	0	0	0	(1)

Examiner said, "Good arguing voice." That was a mistake because it gave specific feedback. It also seemed to encourage the use of a particular voice.

12–14

3. *(for girls)* Thelma <u>disagrees</u> with everything a friend says. Yesterday her friend suggested that they go to a movie on Friday. What do you think Thelma would say?

3. *(for boys)* Theo <u>disagrees</u> with everything a friend says. Yesterday his friend suggested that they go to a movie on Friday. What do you think Theo would say?

Student's response:	Vocabulary	Pragmatics	Item Score	
Disagrees with plan for movie or going on Friday. May (or may not) suggest alternative.	(1)	(1)		
I don't wanna go to the movies.	0	0	0	(1)

Examiner reminded student, "You don't have to use the same voice every time. You can make it be a little different for each one."

4. *(for girls)* Ms. Flynn always gets angry when her class doesn't listen. Her class is really noisy and Ms. Flynn decides to <u>punish</u> the class for not listening. What do you think Ms. Flynn would say?

4. *(for boys)* Mr. Flynn always gets angry when his class doesn't listen. His class is really noisy and Mr. Flynn decides to <u>punish</u> the class for not listening. What do you think Mr. Flynn would say?

Student's response:	Vocabulary	Pragmatics	Item Score	
Uses teacher voice to tell students to quiet down (or some variation) and names a punishment.	(1)	(1)		
Time outs for all of you.	0	0	0	(1)

5. *(for girls)* Rachel wants to <u>politely turn down</u> an invitation to a party she thinks will be boring. What do you think Rachel would say?

5. *(for boys)* Ron wants to <u>politely turn down</u> an invitation to a party he thinks will be boring. What do you think Ron would say?

Student's response:	Vocabulary	Pragmatics	Item Score	
Offers an excuse for not being able to attend in a polite tone, without saying anything about the party being boring.	1	1		
I don't want this invitation (implication)	(0)	(0)	(0)	1

15+

6. *(for girls)* Regina always <u>bullies</u> everyone. All of the kids want her to play soccer, but she will play only if they let her be the goalie. What do you think Regina would say?

6. *(for boys)* Reggie always <u>bullies</u> everyone. All of the kids want him to play soccer, but he will play only if they let him be the goalie. What do you think Reggie would say?

Student's response:	Vocabulary	Pragmatics	Item Score	
Insists on being the goalie in a bullying tone.	(1)	(1)		
I wanna be the goalie.	0	0	0	(1)

This was a challenging one but the decision was to score it as correct because it conveyed the main intent in a bullying tone.

7. *(for girls)* Henry's big sister always <u>orders</u> him to do things for her. She wants him to wash her car. What do you think Henry's big sister would say?

7. *(for boys)* Holly's big brother always <u>orders</u> her to do things for him. He wants her to wash his car. What do you think Holly's big brother would say?

Student's response:	Vocabulary	Pragmatics	Item Score	
Says "wash my car" (or some variation) in a tone that implies ordering. Does not say "please" or offer to pay.	1	(1)		
I want you to wash my car <u>please.</u>	(0)	0	(0)	1

used an ordering tone

8. *(for girls)* Ruth's mother always <u>criticizes</u> everything she does. When Ruth brings home her report card with two As and two Bs, what do you think her mother would say?

8. *(for boys)* Randy's father always <u>criticizes</u> everything he does. When Randy brings home his report card with two As and two Bs, what do you think his father would say?

Student's response:	Vocabulary	Pragmatics	Item Score	
May praise the As, but must convey that the child could have done better.	1	1		
[I don't know what "criticize" means.] /crɛndɪcɪndɪs/	(0)	(0)	(0)	1

9. *(for girls)* Debby always <u>uses hints</u> to get her grandmother to buy her things. Debby is out shopping with her grandmother and sees some boots she wants. What do you think Debby would say?

9. *(for boys)* David always <u>uses hints</u> to get his grandmother to buy him things. David is out shopping with his grandmother and sees some boots he wants. What do you think David would say?

Student's response:	Vocabulary	Pragmatics	Item Score	
Makes comments about how nice the boots are or needing boots but without asking for them directly. (Hinting about the color and shape or location of the boots does not score.)	1	1		
["Hard one."]	(0)	(0)	(0)	1

10. *(for girls)* The talk show host always <u>flatters</u> her guests. She is interviewing an actor. What do you think the talk show host would say?

10. *(for boys)* The talk show host always <u>flatters</u> his guests. He is interviewing an actor. What do you think the talk show host would say?

Student's response:	Vocabulary	Pragmatics	Item Score	
Makes a flattering comment about the guest.	1	1		
Hey, I'm a talk show host.	(0)	(0)	(0)	1

11. *(for girls)* Sarita always <u>encourages</u> her friend to work on her running. Sarita's friend comes in second in a race. What do you think Sarita would say?

11. *(for boys)* Santos always <u>encourages</u> his friend to work on his running. Santos's friend comes in second in a race. What do you think Santos would say?

Student's response:	Vocabulary	Pragmatics	Item Score	
Says something encouraging about continuing to work or coming close or makes a simple praise comment, such as "great job."	(1)	(1)		
Next time you need to run harder.	0	0	0	(1)

[Said in an encouraging voice. Minimal response but met criteria.]

12. *(for girls)* **Sheila always <u>fishes for compliments</u>. She was wearing her new clothes when she met her friend on the way to the school party. What do you think Sheila would say?**

12. *(for boys)* **Shawn always <u>fishes for compliments</u>. He was wearing his new clothes when he met his friend on the way to the school party. What do you think Shawn would say?**

Student's response:	Vocabulary	Pragmatics	Item Score	
Draws attention to self and/or clothes. May ask directly, "How do you like my new clothes?"	1	1		
Aren't you gonna give me a compliment?	(0)	(0)	(0)	1

Examiner wasn't certain how to score this one so gave the last item to be certain to establish the ceiling.

13. *(for girls)* **Nora always <u>sounds really sarcastic</u>. Let's say it rains every weekend all summer. What do you think Nora would say?**

13. *(for boys)* **Noah always <u>sounds really sarcastic</u>. Let's say it rains every weekend all summer. What do you think Noah would say?**

Student's response:	Vocabulary	Pragmatics	Item Score	
Says something ironic about liking all the rain using a sarcastic tone.	1	1		
[I know what sarcastic means, but I don't know how to say it.]	(0)	(0)	(0)	1

Total score: ___6___ / 13

Qualitative observations:

Social Communication (SC) subtest scored for Student 1, a 6-year, 9-month-old boy.

RECAP OF SUBTEST

In the Digit Span Forward (DSF) subtest, the student is asked to repeat a series of digits of advancing length spoken by the examiner at a rate of one per second.

Use as a stand-alone measure: Yes (**Note:** Subtest 14 can be used as a stand-alone measure or in conjunction with Subtest 15. If administered together with Subtest 15, Subtest 14 must be administered immediately before Subtest 15 and in the same session.)

Average time to administer: 3 minutes

Materials: *Examiner Record Form* (p. 36)

Start rule: Start points for age ranges are indicated by arrows.

Basal rule: Scores 1 on all items at any one level (a level is a set of items that all include the same number of digits and are shaded similarly)

Ceiling rule: Scores 0 on all items at any one level

Repetition: No (unless ambient noise interferes)

Probes: None

PRACTICE EXERCISE

To complete this exercise, you will need Track 13 from the Examiner's Practice Workbook Audio Files folder on the *Digital Audio Files* (USB drive) for Student 1, a 6-year, 9-month-old boy with normal language. Listen to the test administration on the audio file and score Student 1's responses using a blank *Examiner Record Form*.

Ask yourself the following questions as you complete the exercise:

1. How are basals and ceilings determined for students age 9 years and older? For students 6–8 years old? What should my next steps be if Student 1 earned a score of 1 on Item 4b?

2. What should I say if a student asks me to repeat an item on this subtest?

ANSWERS

Make your best effort to complete the exercise before you read the following answers:

1. A student who is 9 years or older would need to earn scores of 1 on both Items 2a and 2b (the only two items at Level 2, which is the start point for this age) to achieve a basal. If an older student misses either item, back up and administer both items on Level 1. Students who are 6–8 years old start on Level 1 with Item 1. This then serves as the basal. If Student 1 had earned a score of 1 on Item 4b, you would administer Item 4c and then proceed to Level 5. You would not stop testing until the student missed all of the items at a particular level. In this case, the student actually missed all items on Level 4, so that established the ceiling.

2. If a student asks you to repeat an item on this subtest, you should say, "I'm sorry, I can't repeat that." The only exception is if ambient noise interferes with the student's ability to hear the stimulus.

DIGIT SPAN FORWARD

DSF

Practice Items

Stimulus	Student's response		Stimulus	Student's response
"4–2"	4–2		"8–6"	8–6

Subtest Items

	Item	Stimulus	Student's response	Score		Item	Stimulus	Student's response	Score
6–8	1a.	"5–8–2"	5–8–2	0 (1)		5a.	"7–2–5–8–1–9–4"		0 1
	1b.	"4–1–8"	4–1–8	0 (1)		5b.	"1–7–3–8–6–2–9"		0 1
9+	2a.	"8–2–5–1"	8–2–5–1	0 (1)		5c.	"8–3–9–1–4–1–5"		0 1
	2b.	"6–4–9–3"	6–4–9–3	0 (1)		6a.	"6–1–0–3–9–7–8–1"		0 1
	3a.	"3–8–1–7–2"	3–8–1–7–2	0 (1)		6b.	"2–5–3–1–8–6–4–9"		0 1
	3b.	"7–5–1–4–9"	7–5–1–4–9	0 (1)		6c.	"5–3–4–1–2–9–6–7"		0 1
	4a.	"2–5–9–6–3–8"	2–4–6–9	(0) 1					
	4b.	"9–2–5–8–1–4"	9–2–5–1–4	(0) 1					
	4c.	"6–4–9–7–2–8"	6–4–9–8–2–8	(0) 1					

Ceiling

Total score: __6__ / 15

Qualitative observations:

Digit Span Forward (DSF) subtest scored for Student 1, a 6-year, 9-month-old boy.

In the Digit Span Backward (DSB) subtest, the examiner says a series of digits of advancing length at a rate of one per second. The student must repeat them in backward order.

Use as a stand-alone measure: No (***Note:*** Subtest 14 must be administered immediately prior to Subtest 15 and in the same session.)

Average time to administer: 3 minutes

Materials: *Examiner Record Form* (p. 37)

Start rule: Start points for age ranges are indicated by arrows.

Basal rule: Scores 1 on all items at any one level

Ceiling rule: Scores 0 on all items at any one level

Repetition: No (unless ambient noise interferes)

Probes: None

PRACTICE EXERCISE

To complete this exercise, you will need Track 14 from the Examiner's Practice Workbook Audio Files folder on the *Digital Audio Files* (USB drive) for Student 1, a 6-year, 9-month-old boy with normal language. Listen to the test administration on the audio file and score Student 1's responses using a blank *Examiner Record Form*.

Ask yourself the following questions as you complete the exercise:

1. When does the basal rule change? What does this tell me about the standardization group?

2. What is the ceiling rule?

ANSWERS

Make your best effort to complete the exercise before you read the following answers:

1. Students through the age of 14 years begin with Item 1. This indicates that standardization data showed that students were not predicted to get all Level 1 items correct until they were 15 years old.

2. The ceiling for all students is met when they miss all items at a particular level. Student 1 passed both items at Level 1 but then missed all three items at Level 2.

DIGIT SPAN BACKWARD

DSB

Practice Items

Stimulus	Student's response
"4–2"	2–4 (2–4)

Stimulus	Student's response
"8–6"	6–8 (6–8)

Subtest Items

Item	Stimulus	Student's response	Score	
1a.	"5–8–2"	2–8–5 (2–8–5)	0	(1)
1b.	"4–1–8"	8–1–4 (8–1–4)	0	(1)
1c.	"9–3–7"	7–3–9 (7–3–9)	0	(1)
2a.	"6–4–9–3"	3–9–6–4 (3–9–4–6)	(0)	1
2b.	"8–2–5–1"	1–2–8–9 (1–5–2–8)	(0)	1
2c.	"7–3–1–9"	9–1 (9–1–3–7)	(0)	1
3a.	"3–8–1–7–2"	 (2–7–1–8–3)	0	1
3b.	"7–5–1–4–9"	 (9–4–1–5–7)	0	1

6–14 → (arrow to 1a.)

15+ → (arrow to 2a.)

Ceiling

Item	Stimulus	Student's response	Score	
3c.	"2–9–7–4–8"	 (8–4–7–9–2)	0	1
4a.	"2–5–9–6–3–8"	 (8–3–6–9–5–2)	0	1
4b.	"9–2–5–8–1–4"	 (4–1–8–5–2–9)	0	1
4c.	"6–1–3–2–7–9"	 (9–7–2–3–1–6)	0	1
5a.	"7–2–5–8–1–9–4"	 (4–9–1–8–5–2–7)	0	1
5b.	"1–7–3–8–6–2–9"	 (9–2–6–8–3–7–1)	0	1
5c.	"3–8–1–6–7–2–5"	 (5–2–7–6–1–8–3)	0	1

Total score: 3 / 15

Qualitative observations:

Digit Span Backward (DSB) subtest scored for Student 1, a 6-year, 9-month-old boy.

DSB

Practice Transforming TILLS Raw Scores to Standard Scores

Section I was designed to provide practice in administering and scoring the 15 TILLS subtests to yield raw scores. This section provides practice in how to transform raw scores into standard scores. Raw scores are the scores that are calculated based on the student's responses following rules explained for each subtest in the *TILLS Examiner's Manual* and in Section I of this workbook. Raw scores are transformed into standard scores relative to performance of same-age peers using the tables in the Appendix of the *Examiner's Manual*. Standard scores are based on a scale with a mean of 10 and a standard deviation of 3 so that comparisons may be made across subtests.

Start by using the raw scores for Students 1, 6, and 7 in the three blank Scoring Charts. Use the age-appropriate normative data tables in the Appendix of the *Examiner's Manual* to transform these raw scores into standard scores and percentile ranks. Next, insert the standard scores for specified Identification Core subtests for the student's age in the white cells that match the student's age category (e.g., for 6–7 year-olds: Vocabulary Awareness [VA], Phonemic Awareness [PA], and Nonword Repetition [NWRep]). Answer keys follow the blank Scoring Charts.

DETERMINING THE STUDENT'S AGE

The first example (on p. 70) presents raw scores for the 6-year, 9-month-old boy whose responses have been used for practice in much of this workbook. This example illustrates how to calculate a student's age in years and months. You do this by entering the test date in Year, Month, and Day on the top row and then entering the student's birth date using the same format immediately below. Subtract the bottom number from the top number in the day column first. If the top number is smaller, borrow 30 days from the month column. Then, subtract the bottom number from the top number in the month column. If necessary, borrow 12 months from the year before subtracting. Finally, subtract the student's birth year from the test year. This should establish Student 1's age as 6 years, 9 months. Determine the student's age category based on the student's actual age. Do not round up to the next older age. For example, if a student is 6 years, 11 months, and 29 days, use the normative data tables for students 6;6 through 6;11, not for 7;0 through 7;5.

DETERMINING THE MEAN AND STANDARD DEVIATION

As you complete these exercises, keep in mind that the standard scale used for the individual subtests has a mean of 10 and a standard deviation of 3. Thus, any standard score between 7 and 10 is within 1 standard deviation below the mean for the same-age normative group. Any standard score lower than 7 is more than 1 standard deviation below the mean. Any standard score above 10 is above the mean. A subtest standard score of 13 is 1 standard deviation above the mean. Note that the order of the subtests on the Scoring Chart on the front cover of the *Examiner Record Form* is the same order in which the subtests are administered. This is designed to facilitate data entry.

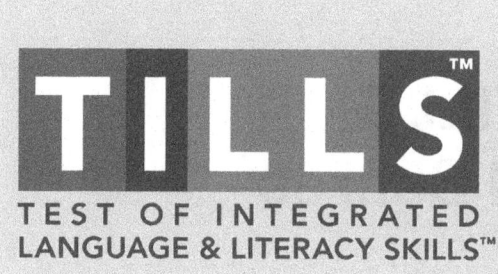

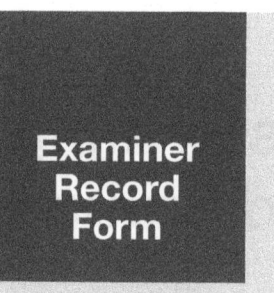

Examiner Record Form

TEST OF INTEGRATED LANGUAGE & LITERACY SKILLS™

CALCULATION OF STUDENT'S AGE
Test date
Year: 2014 Month: 12 Day: 5
Birth date
Year: 2008 Month: 3 Day: 5
Age at test
Year:_____ Month:_____ Day:_____

Student name: _____[Student 1]_____ Grade: _____ School: _____

Scoring Chart

Examiner name: _____

Step 1: Enter raw scores for all subtests administered.

Step 2: Look up the Subtest Standard Scores and Percentile Ranks for the student's age in the *Examiner's Manual* Appendix and enter them in the Subtest Scores section.

Step 3: Copy the Standard Scores into the open white cells on the same rows in the Composite of Subtest Standard Scores section.

Step 4: Copy the Standard Scores into the open white cells in the same rows in the age-appropriate column in the Identification Core Scores section.

Step 5: Enter the Sum of the Subtest Standard Scores in all columns where all subtests have been administered.

Step 6: Look up the Sums of Subtest Standard Scores for the student's age in the *Examiner's Manual* Appendix to find the Standard Scores and Percentile Ranks.

Subtest	Raw Score	Standard Score and TILLS Total	Percentile Rank	Sound/Word Composite Score	Sentence/ Discourse Composite Score	Oral Composite Score	Written Composite Score	Identification Core for 6- to 7-year-olds	Identification Core for 8- to 11-year-olds	Identification Core for 12- to 18-year-olds
		Subtest Scores and TILLS Total		Composite of Subtest Standard Scores				Identification Core Scores		
1 VA	19									
2 PA	13									
3 SR	24									
4 NWRep	20									
5 NWSpell*	6									
6 LC	15									
7 RC*	11									
8 FD	9									
9 DSR	20									
10 NWRead*	8									
11 RF*	64									
12a WE-Disc*	88									
12b WE-Sent*	1.56									
12c WE-Word*	96									
13 SC	6									
14 DSF	6									
15 DSB	3									
Sum of the Subtest Standard Scores										
Standard Scores of the TILLS Total and Composites										
Percentile Ranks for the TILLS Total and Composites										

*Note: For children 6;0–6;5, do not administer the NWSpell, RC, NWRead, RF, and WE subtests.

Key for Subtests: VA = Vocabulary Awareness, PA = Phonemic Awareness, SR = Story Retelling, NWRep = Nonword Repetition, NWSpell = Nonword Spelling, LC = Listening Comprehension, RC = Reading Comprehension, FD = Following Directions, DSR = Delayed Story Retelling, NWRead = Nonword Reading, RF = Reading Fluency, WE-Disc = Written Expression–Discourse Score, WE-Sent = Written Expression–Sentence Score, WE-Word = Written Expression–Word Score, SC = Social Communication, DSF=Digit Span Forward, DSB = Digit Span Backward.

Scoring Chart with raw scores for Student 1, a 6-year, 9-month-old boy.

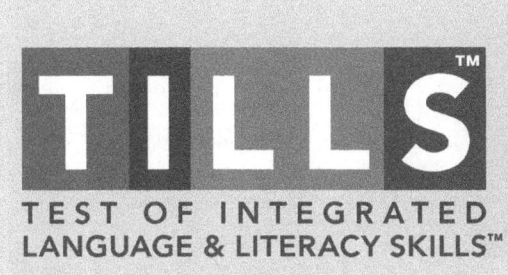
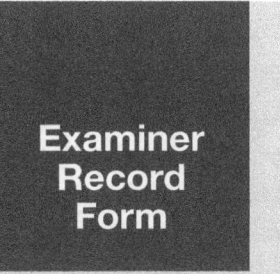

TILLS™

TEST OF INTEGRATED LANGUAGE & LITERACY SKILLS™

Examiner Record Form

CALCULATION OF STUDENT'S AGE		
Test date		
Year: 2014	Month: 12	Day: 5
Birth date		
Year: 2008	Month: 3	Day: 5
Age at test		
Year: 6	Month: 9	Day: 0

Student name: [Student 1] Grade: _____ School: _____

Scoring Chart

Examiner name: _____

Step 1: Enter raw scores for all subtests administered.
Step 2: Look up the Subtest Standard Scores and Percentile Ranks for the student's age in the *Examiner's Manual* Appendix and enter them in the Subtest Scores section.
Step 3: Copy the Standard Scores into the open white cells on the same rows in the Composite of Subtest Standard Scores section.
Step 4: Copy the Standard Scores into the open white cells in the same rows in the age-appropriate column in the Identification Core Scores section.
Step 5: Enter the Sum of the Subtest Standard Scores in all columns where all subtests have been administered.
Step 6: Look up the Sums of Subtest Standard Scores for the student's age in the *Examiner's Manual* Appendix to find the Standard Scores and Percentile Ranks.

Subtest	Raw Score	Standard Score and TILLS Total	Percentile Rank	Sound/Word Composite Score	Sentence/Discourse Composite Score	Oral Composite Score	Written Composite Score	Identification Core for 6- to 7-year-olds	Identification Core for 8- to 11-year-olds	Identification Core for 12- to 18-year-olds
1 VA	19	11	64		11	11		11		
2 PA	13	12	65	12		12		12		
3 SR	24	13	82		13	13				
4 NWRep	20	11	48	11		11		11		
5 NWSpell*	6	13	75	13			13			
6 LC	15	12	65		12	12				
7 RC*	11	13	74		13		13			
8 FD	9	11	63		11	11				
9 DSR	20	12	69		12	12				
10 NWRead*	8	11	66	11			11			
11 RF*	64	11	55	11			11			
12a WE-Disc*	88	13	69		13		13			
12b WE-Sent*	1.56	14	91		14		14			
12c WE-Word*	96	12	66	12			12			
13 SC	6	13	72		13	13				
14 DSF	6	11	65			11				
15 DSB	3	10	59			10				
Sum of the Subtest Standard Scores		203		70	112	116	87	34		
Standard Scores of the TILLS Total and Composites		118		112	119	114	118	109		
Percentile Ranks for the TILLS Total and Composites		86		78	90	80	91	69		

*Note: For children 6;0–6;5, do not administer the NWSpell, RC, NWRead, RF, and WE subtests.

Key for Subtests: VA = Vocabulary Awareness, PA = Phonemic Awareness, SR = Story Retelling, NWRep = Nonword Repetition, NWSpell = Nonword Spelling, LC = Listening Comprehension, RC = Reading Comprehension, FD = Following Directions, DSR = Delayed Story Retelling, NWRead = Nonword Reading, RF = Reading Fluency, WE-Disc = Written Expression–Discourse Score, WE-Sent = Written Expression–Sentence Score, WE-Word = Written Expression–Word Score, SC = Social Communication, DSF=Digit Span Forward, DSB = Digit Span Backward.

Answer Key: Scoring Chart completed for Student 1, a 6-year, 9-month-old boy.

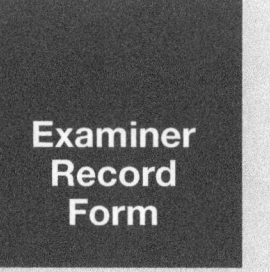

Examiner Record Form

CALCULATION OF STUDENT'S AGE
Test date
Year:_____ Month:_____ Day:_____
Birth date
Year:_____ Month:_____ Day:_____
Age at test
Year: 7 Month: 5 Day: 28

Student name: [Student 6] _____ Grade: _____ School: _____

Scoring Chart

Examiner name: _____

Step 1: Enter raw scores for all subtests administered.

Step 2: Look up the Subtest Standard Scores and Percentile Ranks for the student's age in the *Examiner's Manual* Appendix and enter them in the Subtest Scores section.

Step 3: Copy the Standard Scores into the open white cells on the same rows in the Composite of Subtest Standard Scores section.

Step 4: Copy the Standard Scores into the open white cells in the same rows in the age-appropriate column in the Identification Core Scores section.

Step 5: Enter the Sum of the Subtest Standard Scores in all columns where all subtests have been administered.

Step 6: Look up the Sums of Subtest Standard Scores for the student's age in the *Examiner's Manual* Appendix to find the Standard Scores and Percentile Ranks.

Subtest	Raw Score	Standard Score and TILLS Total	Percentile Rank	Sound/Word Composite Score	Sentence/Discourse Composite Score	Oral Composite Score	Written Composite Score	Identification Core for 6- to 7-year-olds	Identification Core for 8- to 11-year-olds	Identification Core for 12- to 18-year-olds
1 VA	9									
2 PA	2									
3 SR	11									
4 NWRep	17									
5 NWSpell*	3									
6 LC	16									
7 RC*	10									
8 FD	14									
9 DSR	22									
10 NWRead*	2									
11 RF*	64									
12a WE-Disc*	44									
12b WE-Sent*	1.16									
12c WE-Word*	85									
13 SC	3									
14 DSF	3									
15 DSB	2									
Sum of the Subtest Standard Scores										
Standard Scores of the TILLS Total and Composites										
Percentile Ranks for the TILLS Total and Composites										

*Note: For children 6;0–6;5, do not administer the NWSpell, RC, NWRead, RF, and WE subtests.

Key for Subtests: VA = Vocabulary Awareness, PA = Phonemic Awareness, SR = Story Retelling, NWRep = Nonword Repetition, NWSpell = Nonword Spelling, LC = Listening Comprehension, RC = Reading Comprehension, FD = Following Directions, DSR = Delayed Story Retelling, NWRead = Nonword Reading, RF = Reading Fluency, WE-Disc = Written Expression–Discourse Score, WE-Sent = Written Expression–Sentence Score, WE-Word = Written Expression–Word Score, SC = Social Communication, DSF=Digit Span Forward, DSB = Digit Span Backward.

Scoring Chart with raw scores for Student 6, a 7-year, 5-month-old girl.

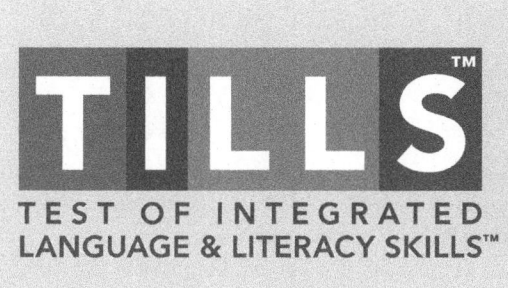

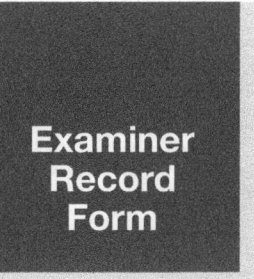

CALCULATION OF STUDENT'S AGE

Test date
Year:_____ Month:_____ Day:_____

Birth date
Year:_____ Month:_____ Day:_____

Age at test
Year: 7 Month: 5 Day: 28

Student name: ___[Student 6]___   Grade: _____ School: _____

Scoring Chart   Examiner name: _____

Step 1: Enter raw scores for all subtests administered.
Step 2: Look up the Subtest Standard Scores and Percentile Ranks for the student's age in the *Examiner's Manual* Appendix and enter them in the Subtest Scores section.
Step 3: Copy the Standard Scores into the open white cells on the same rows in the Composite of Subtest Standard Scores section.
Step 4: Copy the Standard Scores into the open white cells in the same rows in the age-appropriate column in the Identification Core Scores section.
Step 5: Enter the Sum of the Subtest Standard Scores in all columns where all subtests have been administered.
Step 6: Look up the Sums of Subtest Standard Scores for the student's age in the *Examiner's Manual* Appendix to find the Standard Scores and Percentile Ranks.

Subtest	Raw Score	Standard Score and TILLS Total	Percentile Rank	Sound/Word Composite Score	Sentence/ Discourse Composite Score	Oral Composite Score	Written Composite Score	Identification Core for 6- to 7-year-olds	Identification Core for 8- to 11-year-olds	Identification Core for 12- to 18-year-olds
		Subtest Scores and TILLS Total			Composite of Subtest Standard Scores				Identification Core Scores	
1 VA	9	6	6		6	6		6		
2 PA	2	4	4	4		4		4		
3 SR	11	7	16		7	7				
4 NWRep	17	6	5	6		6		6		
5 NWSpell*	3	8	24	8			8			
6 LC	16	11	58		11	11				
7 RC*	10	11	47		11		11			
8 FD	14	15	90		15	15				
9 DSR	22	11	60		11	11				
10 NWRead*	2	5	6	5			5			
11 RF*	64	10	34	10			10			
12a WE-Disc*	44	8	27		8		8			
12b WE-Sent*	1.16	9	47		9		9			
12c WE-Word*	85	9	18	9			9			
13 SC	3	8	18		8	8				
14 DSF	3	6	2			6				
15 DSB	2	9	24			9				
Sum of the Subtest Standard Scores		143		42	86	83	60	16		
Standard Scores of the TILLS Total and Composites		87		79	97	87	90	69		
Percentile Ranks for the TILLS Total and Composites		19		5	38	20	18	2		

*Note: For children 6;0–6;5, do not administer the NWSpell, RC, NWRead, RF, and WE subtests.

Key for Subtests: VA = Vocabulary Awareness, PA = Phonemic Awareness, SR = Story Retelling, NWRep = Nonword Repetition, NWSpell = Nonword Spelling, LC = Listening Comprehension, RC = Reading Comprehension, FD = Following Directions, DSR = Delayed Story Retelling, NWRead = Nonword Reading, RF = Reading Fluency, WE-Disc = Written Expression–Discourse Score, WE-Sent = Written Expression–Sentence Score, WE-Word = Written Expression–Word Score, SC = Social Communication, DSF=Digit Span Forward, DSB = Digit Span Backward.

Answer Key: Scoring Chart completed for Student 6, a 7-year, 5-month-old girl.

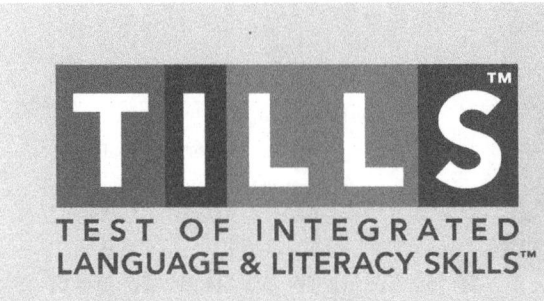

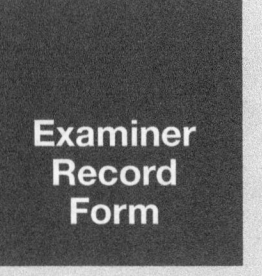

Examiner Record Form

CALCULATION OF STUDENT'S AGE

Test date
Year:_____ Month:_____ Day:_____

Birth date
Year:_____ Month:_____ Day:_____

Age at test
Year: 13 Month: 7 Day:_____

Student name: [Student 7] Grade: _____ School: _____

Scoring Chart

Examiner name: _____

Step 1: Enter raw scores for all subtests administered.
Step 2: Look up the Subtest Standard Scores and Percentile Ranks for the student's age in the *Examiner's Manual* Appendix and enter them in the Subtest Scores section.
Step 3: Copy the Standard Scores into the open white cells on the same rows in the Composite of Subtest Standard Scores section.
Step 4: Copy the Standard Scores into the open white cells in the same rows in the age-appropriate column in the Identification Core Scores section.
Step 5: Enter the Sum of the Subtest Standard Scores in all columns where all subtests have been administered.
Step 6: Look up the Sums of Subtest Standard Scores for the student's age in the *Examiner's Manual* Appendix to find the Standard Scores and Percentile Ranks.

Subtest	Raw Score	Standard Score and TILLS Total	Percentile Rank	Sound/Word Composite Score	Sentence/Discourse Composite Score	Oral Composite Score	Written Composite Score	Identification Core for 6- to 7-year-olds	Identification Core for 8- to 11-year-olds	Identification Core for 12- to 18-year-olds
1 VA	31									
2 PA	18									
3 SR	11									
4 NWRep	24									
5 NWSpell*	12									
6 LC	15									
7 RC*	11									
8 FD	9									
9 DSR	16									
10 NWRead*	16									
11 RF*	130									
12a WE-Disc*	77									
12b WE-Sent*	2.67									
12c WE-Word*	92									
13 SC	6									
14 DSF	7									
15 DSB	3									
Sum of the Subtest Standard Scores										
Standard Scores of the TILLS Total and Composites										
Percentile Ranks for the TILLS Total and Composites										

*Note: For children 6;0–6;5, do not administer the NWSpell, RC, NWRead, RF, and WE subtests.

Key for Subtests: VA = Vocabulary Awareness, PA = Phonemic Awareness, SR = Story Retelling, NWRep = Nonword Repetition, NWSpell = Nonword Spelling, LC = Listening Comprehension, RC = Reading Comprehension, FD = Following Directions, DSR = Delayed Story Retelling, NWRead = Nonword Reading, RF = Reading Fluency, WE-Disc = Written Expression–Discourse Score, WE-Sent = Written Expression–Sentence Score, WE-Word = Written Expression–Word Score, SC = Social Communication, DSF=Digit Span Forward, DSB = Digit Span Backward.

Scoring Chart with raw scores for Student 7, a 13-year-old boy.

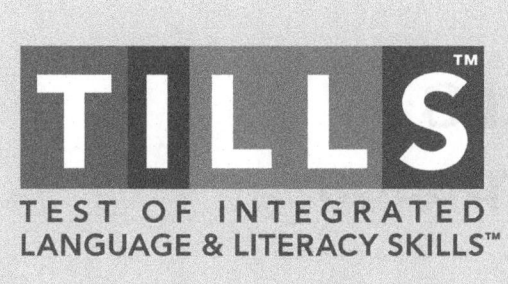 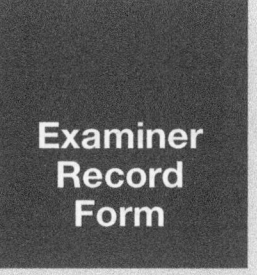

CALCULATION OF STUDENT'S AGE

Test date
Year:_____ Month:_____ Day:_____

Birth date
Year:_____ Month:_____ Day:_____

Age at test
Year: 13 Month: 7 Day:_____

Student name: __[Student 7]_____ Grade: _____ School: _____

Scoring Chart

Examiner name: _____

Step 1: Enter raw scores for all subtests administered.
Step 2: Look up the Subtest Standard Scores and Percentile Ranks for the student's age in the *Examiner's Manual* Appendix and enter them in the Subtest Scores section.
Step 3: Copy the Standard Scores into the open white cells on the same rows in the Composite of Subtest Standard Scores section.
Step 4: Copy the Standard Scores into the open white cells in the same rows in the age-appropriate column in the Identification Core Scores section.
Step 5: Enter the Sum of the Subtest Standard Scores in all columns where all subtests have been administered.
Step 6: Look up the Sums of Subtest Standard Scores for the student's age in the *Examiner's Manual* Appendix to find the Standard Scores and Percentile Ranks.

Subtest	Raw Score	Standard Score and TILLS Total	Percentile Rank	Sound/Word Composite Score	Sentence/ Discourse Composite Score	Oral Composite Score	Written Composite Score	Identification Core for 6- to 7-year-olds	Identification Core for 8- to 11-year-olds	Identification Core for 12- to 18-year-olds
1 VA	31	5	4		5	5				
2 PA	18	8	16	8		8				8
3 SR	11	4	3		4	4				
4 NWRep	24	14	82	14		14				
5 NWSpell*	12	8	22	8			8			8
6 LC	15	5	4		5	5				
7 RC*	11	2	2		2		2			2
8 FD	9	5	5		5	5				
9 DSR	16	5	9		5	5				
10 NWRead*	16	8	12	8			8			
11 RF*	130	12	55	12			12			12
12a WE-Disc*	77	8	17		8		8			
12b WE-Sent*	2.67	12	82		12		12			
12c WE-Word*	92	1	1	1			1			1
13 SC	6	2	0		2	2				
14 DSF	7	7	16			7				
15 DSB	3	6	6			6				
Sum of the Subtest Standard Scores		112		51	48	61	51			31
Standard Scores of the TILLS Total and Composites		66		88	57	64	76			68
Percentile Ranks for the TILLS Total and Composites		2		21	0	0	7			4

*Note: For children 6;0–6;5, do not administer the NWSpell, RC, NWRead, RF, and WE subtests.
Key for Subtests: VA = Vocabulary Awareness, PA = Phonemic Awareness, SR = Story Retelling, NWRep = Nonword Repetition, NWSpell = Nonword Spelling, LC = Listening Comprehension, RC = Reading Comprehension, FD = Following Directions, DSR = Delayed Story Retelling, NWRead = Nonword Reading, RF = Reading Fluency, WE-Disc = Written Expression–Discourse Score, WE-Sent = Written Expression–Sentence Score, WE-Word = Written Expression–Word Score, SC = Social Communication, DSF=Digit Span Forward, DSB = Digit Span Backward.

Answer Key: Scoring Chart completed for Student 7, a 13-year-old boy.

Practice Interpreting TILLS Results for Its Three Purposes

The three validated purposes of the TILLS are 1) to identify language and literacy disorders, 2) to document patterns of relative strengths and weaknesses, and 3) to track changes in language and literacy skills over time (periods of 6 months or more). To complete these practice exercises, you will need to refer to Chapter 3 and the Appendix in the *TILLS Examiner's Manual*. The steps for interpreting TILLS results for identifying disorder and tracking change over time are printed on the inside back cover of the *TILLS Examiner Record Form,* where you will enter the data. The basic steps for documenting strengths and weaknesses are printed on the back cover.

These exercises will help strengthen your skills at manually scoring the Identification Chart (for Purpose 1), the Profile Chart (for Purpose 2), and the Tracking Chart (for Purpose 3). It is important to understand *how* these scores are calculated so that you become familiar with interpreting the information they provide. After completing these exercises, you may choose to use the *Easy-Score*™ tool to obtain the same information in less time. Completing the exercises first, however, will give you a better understanding of what the scores mean.

The *TILLS Easy-Score*™ tool, available from Brookes Publishing, can help you complete all of the scoring charts on the *Examiner Record Form.* After you enter the student's birthdate, test date, and raw scores for the individual subtests, *Easy-Score* automatically completes the rest of a Scoring Chart like the one on the cover of the *Examiner Record Form.* It does so by filling in the age-appropriate standard scores, percentile ranks, composite scores, and identification core score for the student. It also generates report-ready text for skills tested. Using the Scoring Chart information, *Easy-Score* can then complete the Identification Chart (showing the student's result compared to the age-appropriate cut score) and the Profile Chart (graphing the student's relative strengths and weaknesses across the subtests and plotting confidence intervals). If you have two administrations of the TILLS for the same student given 6 months or more apart, *Easy-Score* can also fill in the Tracking Chart to show where true change is identified. (For more information on *Easy-Score,* visit www.brookes publishing.com/tills.)

PURPOSE 1: TO IDENTIFY LANGUAGE AND LITERACY DISORDERS

As specified at the top of the inside back cover of the *Examiner Record Form,* identifying language and literacy disorders involves performing the following steps:

Step 1: Enter the Sum of the Subtest Standard Scores from the age-appropriate column in the Identification Core Score section from the Scoring Chart on the front cover of the *Examiner Record Form.*

Step 2: Compare this score to the appropriate age band and cut score. Check the decision box to the right of the table.

Practice Exercise

To complete these practice exercises, use the standard score data you compiled for Practice Transforming TILLS Raw Scores to Standard Scores for Students 1, 6, and 7 (pp. 70–75). This will allow you to complete Step 1 for all 3 students by entering the Identification Core Sum in the appropriate box on the blank scoring forms on the following page. Then, complete Step 2 for each of the 3 students by comparing the Identification Core scores to the cut scores for the students' ages and answering the identification question Yes or No. Make your best effort to complete the exercise before proceeding.

Identification Chart

Purpose: To identify language and literacy disorders

Step 1: Enter the Sum of the Subtest Standard Scores from the age-appropriate column for the Identification Core Score section from the Scoring Chart of the front cover of this *Examiner Record Form.*

Step 2: Compare this score to the appropriate age band and cut score. Check the decision box to the right of the table.

Age Band	Sum of Identification Core Standard Scores	Cut Score	Sensitivity	Specificity	Decision: Is the Identification Core composite less than the cut score?
6–7 years		24	84	84	❐ Yes — This score is consistent with the presence of a language/literacy disorder. ❐ No — This score is not consistent with the presence of a language/literacy disorder.
8–11 years		34	88	85	
12–18 years		42	86	90	

Note: The confidence in the diagnostic decision is related to the sensitivity and specificity values for the student's age. Please refer to Chapter 2 of the *Technical Manual* for more information. Be sure to use the *Sum* of the Identification Core Standard Scores and *not* the Standard Score of the Identification Core Composite for comparison to the cut score.

Blank practice form to use for Student 1.

Identification Chart

Purpose: To identify language and literacy disorders

Step 1: Enter the Sum of the Subtest Standard Scores from the age-appropriate column for the Identification Core Score section from the Scoring Chart of the front cover of this *Examiner Record Form.*

Step 2: Compare this score to the appropriate age band and cut score. Check the decision box to the right of the table.

Age Band	Sum of Identification Core Standard Scores	Cut Score	Sensitivity	Specificity	Decision: Is the Identification Core composite less than the cut score?
6–7 years		24	84	84	❐ Yes — This score is consistent with the presence of a language/literacy disorder. ❐ No — This score is not consistent with the presence of a language/literacy disorder.
8–11 years		34	88	85	
12–18 years		42	86	90	

Note: The confidence in the diagnostic decision is related to the sensitivity and specificity values for the student's age. Please refer to Chapter 2 of the *Technical Manual* for more information. Be sure to use the *Sum* of the Identification Core Standard Scores and *not* the Standard Score of the Identification Core Composite for comparison to the cut score.

Blank practice form to use for Student 6.

Identification Chart

Purpose: To identify language and literacy disorders

Step 1: Enter the Sum of the Subtest Standard Scores from the age-appropriate column for the Identification Core Score section from the Scoring Chart of the front cover of this *Examiner Record Form.*

Step 2: Compare this score to the appropriate age band and cut score. Check the decision box to the right of the table.

Age Band	Sum of Identification Core Standard Scores	Cut Score	Sensitivity	Specificity	Decision: Is the Identification Core composite less than the cut score?
6–7 years		24	84	84	❐ Yes — This score is consistent with the presence of a language/literacy disorder. ❐ No — This score is not consistent with the presence of a language/literacy disorder.
8–11 years		34	88	85	
12–18 years		42	86	90	

Note: The confidence in the diagnostic decision is related to the sensitivity and specificity values for the student's age. Please refer to Chapter 2 of the *Technical Manual* for more information. Be sure to use the *Sum* of the Identification Core Standard Scores and *not* the Standard Score of the Identification Core Composite for comparison to the cut score.

Blank practice form to use for Student 7.

Blank Identification Charts to be completed for Students 1, 6, and 7.

Identification Chart

Purpose: To identify language and literacy disorders

Step 1: Enter the Sum of the Subtest Standard Scores from the age-appropriate column for the Identification Core Score section from the Scoring Chart of the front cover of this *Examiner Record Form.*

Step 2: Compare this score to the appropriate age band and cut score. Check the decision box to the right of the table.

Age Band	Sum of Identification Core Standard Scores	Cut Score	Sensitivity	Specificity	Decision: Is the Identification Core composite less than the cut score?
6–7 years	34	24	84	84	☐ Yes ☒ No
8–11 years		34	88	85	This score is consistent with the presence of a language/ literacy disorder. / This score is not consistent with the presence of a language/ literacy disorder.
12–18 years		42	86	90	

Note: The confidence in the diagnostic decision is related to the sensitivity and specificity values for the student's age. Please refer to Chapter 2 of the *Technical Manual* for more information. Be sure to use the *Sum* of the Identification Core Standard Scores and *not* the Standard Score of the Identification Core Composite for comparison to the cut score.

Answer Key: Identification Chart completed for Student 1, a 6-year, 9-month-old boy.

Identification Chart

Purpose: To identify language and literacy disorders

Step 1: Enter the Sum of the Subtest Standard Scores from the age-appropriate column for the Identification Core Score section from the Scoring Chart of the front cover of this *Examiner Record Form.*

Step 2: Compare this score to the appropriate age band and cut score. Check the decision box to the right of the table.

Age Band	Sum of Identification Core Standard Scores	Cut Score	Sensitivity	Specificity	Decision: Is the Identification Core composite less than the cut score?
6–7 years	16	24	84	84	☒ Yes ☐ No
8–11 years		34	88	85	This score is consistent with the presence of a language/ literacy disorder. / This score is not consistent with the presence of a language/ literacy disorder.
12–18 years		42	86	90	

Note: The confidence in the diagnostic decision is related to the sensitivity and specificity values for the student's age. Please refer to Chapter 2 of the *Technical Manual* for more information. Be sure to use the *Sum* of the Identification Core Standard Scores and *not* the Standard Score of the Identification Core Composite for comparison to the cut score.

Answer Key: Identification Chart completed for Student 6, a 7-year, 5-month-old girl.

Identification Chart

Purpose: To identify language and literacy disorders

Step 1: Enter the Sum of the Subtest Standard Scores from the age-appropriate column for the Identification Core Score section from the Scoring Chart of the front cover of this *Examiner Record Form.*

Step 2: Compare this score to the appropriate age band and cut score. Check the decision box to the right of the table.

Age Band	Sum of Identification Core Standard Scores	Cut Score	Sensitivity	Specificity	Decision: Is the Identification Core composite less than the cut score?
6–7 years		24	84	84	☒ Yes ☐ No
8–11 years		34	88	85	This score is consistent with the presence of a language/ literacy disorder. / This score is not consistent with the presence of a language/ literacy disorder.
12–18 years	31	42	86	90	

Note: The confidence in the diagnostic decision is related to the sensitivity and specificity values for the student's age. Please refer to Chapter 2 of the *Technical Manual* for more information. Be sure to use the *Sum* of the Identification Core Standard Scores and *not* the Standard Score of the Identification Core Composite for comparison to the cut score.

Answer Key: Identification Chart completed for Student 7, a 13-year-old boy.

Answers

The results for Student 1, a 6-year, 9-month old boy, shown on page 71 clearly indicate no evidence of language and literacy disorder. His Identification Core composite sum of the standard score of 34 is above the cut score of 24 and consistent with his normal language developmental history.

The Identification Core composite sum of the standard score of 16 for the 7-year, 5-month-old girl is lower than the cut score, supporting the identification of a language and literacy disorder.

The Identification Core composite sum of the standard score of 31 for Student 7, a 13-year-old boy, is lower than the cut score of 42 and thus is consistent with his existing diagnosis of language learning disability.

PURPOSE 2: TO DOCUMENT PATTERNS OF RELATIVE STRENGTHS AND WEAKNESSES

Whether or not a student is identified as having a disorder, it can be helpful to consider patterns of strengths and weaknesses as represented by his or her standard scores on the TILLS. This is the second purpose of the TILLS. As specified in the Profile Chart on the back cover of the *Examiner Record Form,* documenting patterns of relative strengths and weaknesses of language and literacy disorders involves performing the following steps:

Step 1: For each subtest administered, enter the Standard Score from the Scoring Chart (on the front cover) in the white cell at the top of the corresponding subtest column in the Profile Chart.

Step 2: Mark an X over the dot for the corresponding score in the column.

Step 3: Draw a vertical line from the X to the horizontal line representing the mean in the chart (at standard score 10).

Practice Exercise

This exercise involves plotting the standard scores for Students 1, 6, and 7 using the data you compiled for Practice Transforming TILLS Raw Scores to Standard Scores (Section IIA). Enter the standard scores from these charts onto the blank Profile Charts included on the next page. Make your best effort to complete the exercise before proceeding.

Answers

The Profile Chart for Student 1, a 6-year, 9-month-old boy, shows subtest scores all above the mean. This student is clearly performing above average on the language and literacy skills assessed with the TILLS.

The Profile Chart for Student 6, a 7-year, 5-month-old girl, shows a mixture of strengths and weaknesses. When considering the features of this profile, the assessment team might observe that the student shows relative strengths in sentence/discourse-level skills and weaknesses in sound/word-level skills, except that her initial story retelling skills were weak.

When considering the TILLS profile for Student 7, a 13-year-old boy, the most striking finding is that all of his oral language sentence/discourse-level abilities fall more than 1 standard deviation below the mean. He shows particular strengths for repeating nonwords and reading real words fluently. However, his spelling of real words is extremely low, as is his vocabulary awareness. This student's team could also observe that reading comprehension is even lower than listening comprehension despite the fact that his reading fluency score is above average.

Chart 1

		Oral Language										Written Language						
		Sound/Word Level				Sentence/Discourse Level						Sound/Word Level				Sent/Disc Level		
		PA	NW Rep	DSF	DSB	VA	LC	FD	SR	DSR	SC	NW Read	RF	NW Spell	WE-Word	RC	WE-Disc	WE-Sent
	Standard Score																	
+2 SD	16–19																	
	15																	
	14																	
+1 SD	13																	
	12																	
	11																	
Mean	10																	
	9																	
	8																	
−1 SD	7																	
	6																	
	5																	
−2 SD	4																	
	3																	
	2																	
−3 SD	1																	
	0																	

Chart 2

		Oral Language										Written Language						
		Sound/Word Level				Sentence/Discourse Level						Sound/Word Level				Sent/Disc Level		
		PA	NW Rep	DSF	DSB	VA	LC	FD	SR	DSR	SC	NW Read	RF	NW Spell	WE-Word	RC	WE-Disc	WE-Sent
	Standard Score																	
+2 SD	16–19																	
	15																	
	14																	
+1 SD	13																	
	12																	
	11																	
Mean	10																	
	9																	
	8																	
−1 SD	7																	
	6																	
	5																	
−2 SD	4																	
	3																	
	2																	
−3 SD	1																	
	0																	

Chart 3

		Oral Language										Written Language						
		Sound/Word Level				Sentence/Discourse Level						Sound/Word Level				Sent/Disc Level		
		PA	NW Rep	DSF	DSB	VA	LC	FD	SR	DSR	SC	NW Read	RF	NW Spell	WE-Word	RC	WE-Disc	WE-Sent
	Standard Score																	
+2 SD	16–19																	
	15																	
	14																	
+1 SD	13																	
	12																	
	11																	
Mean	10																	
	9																	
	8																	
−1 SD	7																	
	6																	
	5																	
−2 SD	4																	
	3																	
	2																	
−3 SD	1																	
	0																	

Blank Profile Charts to be completed for Students 1, 6, and 7

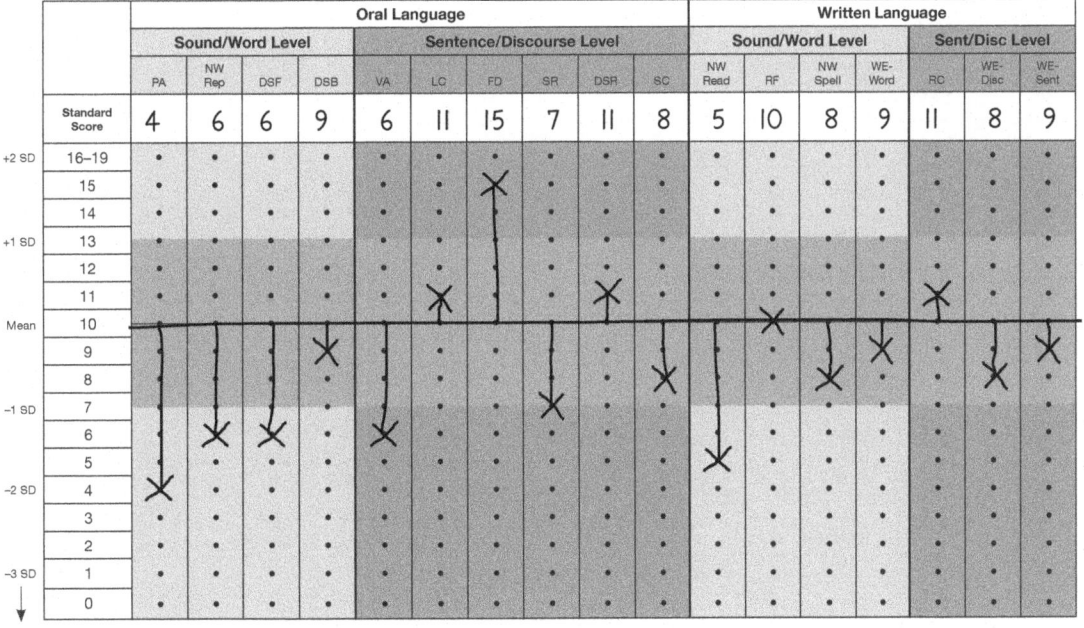

Answer Key: Profile Chart completed for Student 1, a 6-year, 9-month-old boy.

Answer Key: Profile Chart completed for Student 6, a 7-year, 5-month-old girl.

		Oral Language										Written Language						
		Sound/Word Level				Sentence/Discourse Level						Sound/Word Level				Sent/Disc Level		
		PA	NW Rep	DSF	DSB	VA	LC	FD	SR	DSR	SC	NW Read	RF	NW Spell	WE-Word	RC	WE-Disc	WE-Sent
	Standard Score	8	14	7	6	5	5	5	4	5	2	8	12	8	1	2	8	12
+2 SD	16–19																	
	15																	
	14		X															
+1 SD	13																	
	12												X					X
	11																	
Mean	10																	
	9																	
	8	X										X		X			X	
–1 SD	7			X														
	6				X													
	5					X	X	X		X								
–2 SD	4								X									
	3																	
	2										X					X		
–3 SD	1														X			
↓	0																	

Answer Key: Profile Chart completed for Student 7, a 13-year-old boy.

PURPOSE 3: TO TRACK CHANGES IN LANGUAGE AND LITERACY SKILLS OVER TIME

The third purpose of the TILLS is to track change over time. The tracking purpose can be accomplished if a period of at least 6 months (to prevent learning the test) separates the original test from the retest. Meeting the tracking purpose involves performing the following five steps:

Step 1: Enter the standard scores obtained at Test Time 1 (from an earlier administration of the TILLS) and Test Time 2 (from the current administration) for each subtest administered.

Step 2: Subtract standard scores earned at Time 1 from scores earned at Time 2 to calculate differences.

Step 3: Compare the absolute values of the differences (i.e., ignoring whether they are positive or negative) to the True Change Interval values. (These represent values for the 68% confidence interval; values for the 90% confidence interval are reported in the Appendix of the *Examiner's Manual*.)

Step 4: If the absolute value of the difference for a subtest is larger than the True Change Interval, enter "yes" (or Y) under Change Decision. If not, enter "no" (or N). If yes, use a sign (+ or –) to indicate whether the difference is positive or negative.

Practice Exercise

The practice material for this workbook exercise was generated when a 7-year, 5-month-old girl was retested 2 years later. At that point, this student was 9 years, 3 months old. To accomplish the third TILLS purpose of determining whether significant change has occurred in the student's performance relative to peers, complete the following Tracking Chart. Make your best effort to complete the exercise before proceeding.

Tracking Chart

Purpose: To track changes in language and literacy skills over time

Step 1: Enter the Standard Score obtained at Test Time 1 (from an earlier administration of the TILLS) and Test Time 2 (from the current administration) for each subtest administered.

Step 2: Subtract standard scores earned at Time 1 from scores earned at Time 2 to calculate differences.

Step 3: Compare the absolute values of the differences (i.e., ignoring whether they are positive or negative) to the True Change Interval values. (These represent values for the 68% confidence interval; values for the 90% confidence interval are reported in the Appendix of the *Examiner's Manual*.)

Step 4: If the absolute value of the difference for a subtest is larger than the True Change Interval, enter "yes" (or Y) under Change Decision. If not, enter "no" (or N). If yes, add a sign (+ or –) to indicate whether the difference is positive or negative.

DATE OF TEST		AGE OF STUDENT		
Test Time 2: 10/1/15		9 yrs	3 mos	
Test Time 1: 12/5/13		7 yrs	5 mos	
Time between tests: 21 mos		(minimum 6 months)		

	Sub-test	Standard Score Time 2	Standard Score Time 1	Difference	True Change Interval	Change Decision (yes/no)	Sub-test	Standard Score Time 2	Standard Score Time 1	Difference	True Change Interval	Change Decision (yes/no)
		Oral Language						**Written Language**				
Sound/Word Level	PA	9	4		2		NW Read	2	5		1	
	NW Rep	8	6		2		RF	7	10		2	
	DSF	7	6		2		NW Spell	6	8		1	
	DSB	4	9		2		WE-Word	7	9		2	
Sent/Disc Level	VA	7	6		1		RC	9	11		2	
	LC	11	11		2		WE-Disc	11	8		1	
	FD	10	15		2		WE-Sent	9	9		1	
	SR	7	7		2							
	DSR	6	11		2							
	SC	7	8		2							

Tracking Chart with Time 2 and Time 1 scores entered for Student 6, now a 9-year, 3-month-old girl.

Answers

This girl, who was tested first at age 7 years, 5 months and then again at age 9 years, 3 months, showed significant increasing difficulties relative to same-age peers on the second TILLS testing in a number of areas. Although she improved her sound/word-level skills in the area of phonemic awareness, skills declined compared to norms on several subtests in the written modality. Of equal concern, some of her oral language sentence/discourse-level skills (Following Directions and Delayed Story Retelling) also declined relative to her chronological age peers. Beyond formal testing, her clinician reported that this student was now refusing to attempt reading and writing tasks. At this point, her multidisciplinary evaluation team used the TILLS data and other input to find her eligible for special education on the basis of having a language-based learning disability.

Tracking Chart

Purpose: To track changes in language and literacy skills over time

Step 1: Enter the Standard Score obtained at Test Time 1 (from an earlier administration of the TILLS) and Test Time 2 (from the current administration) for each subtest administered.

Step 2: Subtract standard scores earned at Time 1 from scores earned at Time 2 to calculate differences.

Step 3: Compare the absolute values of the differences (i.e., ignoring whether they are positive or negative) to the True Change Interval values. (These represent values for the 68% confidence interval; values for the 90% confidence interval are reported in the Appendix of the *Examiner's Manual*.)

Step 4: If the absolute value of the difference for a subtest is larger than the True Change Interval, enter "yes" (or Y) under Change Decision. If not, enter "no" (or N). If yes, add a sign (+ or –) to indicate whether the difference is positive or negative.

DATE OF TEST		AGE OF STUDENT		
Test Time 2: 10/1/15		9 yrs	3 mos	
Test Time 1: 12/5/13		7 yrs	5 mos	
Time between tests: 21 mos			*(minimum 6 months)*	

		Oral Language					Written Language					
	Sub-test	Standard Score Time 2	Standard Score Time 1	Difference	True Change Interval	Change Decision (yes/no)	Sub-test	Standard Score Time 2	Standard Score Time 1	Difference	True Change Interval	Change Decision (yes/no)
Sound/Word Level	PA	9	4	+5	2	Y+	NW Read	2	5	–3	1	Y–
	NW Rep	8	6	+2	2	N	RF	7	10	–3	2	Y–
	DSF	7	6	+1	2	N	NW Spell	6	8	–2	1	Y–
	DSB	4	9	–5	2	Y–	WE-Word	7	9	–2	2	N
Sent/Disc Level	VA	7	6	+1	1	N	RC	9	11	–2	2	N
	LC	11	11	0	2	N	WE-Disc	11	8	+3	1	Y+
	FD	10	15	–5	2	Y–	WE-Sent	9	9	0	1	N
	SR	7	7	0	2	N						
	DSR	6	11	–5	2	Y–						
	SC	7	8	–1	2	N						

Answer Key: Differences and Change Decisions for Student 6 from Time 1 to Time 2.

Tutorial on Grammar and T-Unit Division for the Written Expression Subtest

OVERVIEW OF WRITTEN EXPRESSION (WE) TASK AND SCORING

To complete the Written Expression (WE) subtest, students must rewrite the set of facts they read aloud for the Reading Fluency (RF) subtest to tell the same story but in a way that sounds less choppy and more interesting. The facts are printed on a page in the *TILLS Stimulus Book* as a series of short kernel sentences (essentially a noun phrase + a verb phrase). The four age-appropriate stories must be read initially as part of the RF subtest. If the student has difficulty reading any words in the facts, the examiner reads them aloud immediately before asking the student to rewrite the story. The age-appropriate stories (with *Stimulus Book* page numbers) are as follows:

- Story A (ages 6;6–7;11) "The Class Pet" (p. 69)

- Story B (ages 8;0–10;11) "The Principal's Daughter" (p. 71)

- Story C (ages 11;0–13;11) "When the School Closed" (p. 73)

- Story D (ages 14;0–18;11) "The Building" (p. 75)

The WE subtest is essentially a sentence-combining task. That is, students are asked to put the facts from their story together in a way that sounds less choppy and more interesting. They are shown a model of how to do this for a short set of eight facts that tell a story about "The Little Dog" (p. 77 in the *Stimulus Book*) along with an example in the *Student Response Form* (p. 7) of how someone put those facts together. The student is not explicitly told how to do this. The only prompt is for the student to put the facts for his or her story together in a way that sounds less choppy and more interesting.

Students rewrite the facts in their own story on page 8 of the *Student Response Form*. To do so requires students to understand facts of the story and how they are related. Students then must formulate complex sentence structures to convey the same facts (content units) and retell the story in writing, using sentences that are grammatically correct and composed of correctly spelled words.

These integrated skills are assessed by calculating three quantitative measures to characterize the student's written expression abilities at three language levels:

- Written Expression–Discourse score (WE-Disc)

- Written Expression–Sentence score (WE-Sent)

- Written Expression–Word score (WE-Word)

This task and scoring methods for assessing the three levels were selected based on extensive pilot research for the TILLS as performing the best for differentiating students by age and disability group.

These training materials are modified from materials developed originally by Michelle DeMaagd-Slager (2011) for her master's thesis research completed at Western Michigan University.

Written Expression–Discourse Score (WE-Disc)

Calculate the Written Expression–Discourse score (WE-Disc) as the percentage of content units included in the student's rewritten story out of the total possible content units. If a student has written a fact that corresponds to the underlined words in a content unit in the age-appropriate story in the *Examiner's Record Form,* circle 1. To earn credit, the student must convey the content specified, but he or she may convey the same content in different words. Next, count the total number of scores of 1 and divide that total by the number of possible content units in the story. Multiply by 100 to calculate the percentage. Example Story A ("The Class Pet") lists 16 possible content units.

WRITTEN EXPRESSION CONTENT UNITS SCORING FORM
Story A: "The Class Pet" (p. 69)

1. The <u>class</u> has a <u>pet</u>.	0	(1)	9. The <u>door</u> was open.	0	(1)
2. It is a <u>hamster</u>.	0	(1)	10. The children <u>looked</u>.	(0)	1
3. The hamster has <u>spots</u>.	0	(1)	11. The children <u>found</u> him.	0	(1)
4. Some are <u>brown</u>.	0	(1)	12. They <u>put him back</u>.	0	(1)
5. Some are <u>white</u>.	0	(1)	13. They put him in the <u>cage</u>.	(0)	1
6. It <u>got out</u>.	0	(1)	14. They closed the <u>door</u>.	(0)	1
7. It was one day <u>last week</u>.	0	(1)	15. He found a <u>corner</u>.	0	(1)
8. The cage was <u>open</u>.	0	(1)	16. He went to <u>sleep</u>.	0	(1)
			Content Units total		13 /16

This student included 13 of the 16 content units. This corresponds to a WE-Disc score of 81%, which is calculated as follows:

$$\frac{13 \text{ content units included}}{16 \text{ possible}} \times 100 = 81.25\% \text{ (rounds to 81\%)}$$

Written Expression–Sentence Score (WE-Sent)

Calculate Written Expression–Sentence score (WE-Sent) as the total number of content units included by the student divided by the number of T-units the student uses to express that content. (See the T-unit tutorial, which starts on p. 90.) Carry the ratio to two decimal points. To arrive at this score, start by making a slash mark after each T-unit. Count these slash marks to yield the total number of T-units. Then, divide the total number of content units by the total number of T-units. For example, a student might copy Story A exactly. Story A has 16 possible content units. Copying would yield 16 T-units, leading to a WE-Sent score of 1.00.

$$\frac{16 \text{ content units}}{16 \text{ T-units}} = 1.00$$

In another example, a student might demonstrate higher-level sentence-combining skills by incorporating all 16 content units into 5 T-units. In this case, the WE-Sent score would be calculated as follows:

$$\frac{16 \text{ content units}}{5 \text{ T-units}} = 3.20$$

As a third example, it would be possible to earn a score of less than 1.00 if the student adds information that is not in the original story, yielding more T-units than content units. An example would be 8 content units divided by 10 T-units (2 of which added content not in the original story), yielding a WE-Sent score of .80.

$$\frac{8 \text{ content units}}{10 \text{ T-units}} = .80$$

In the example Story A, you can see that the examiner put a slash mark after each T-unit, and there are six slash marks corresponding to six T-units. The most challenging decision was how to mark "It was one day last week it got out." One could argue that this construction should be coded as two separate T-units, "It was one day last week" and "It got out." The examiner decided to code this example as 1 T-unit, however, following the general principle to give credit when in doubt. In this case, the subordinating conjunction could be understood, as in, "It was one day last week [that] it got out." There are 16 possible content units in Story A (see the *Examiner Record Form* for the total possible content units for each story). As noted previously, this student incorporated 13 of them. Thus, the student's WE-Sent score is calculated as follows:

$$\frac{13 \text{ content units}}{6 \text{ T-units}} = 2.17$$

Written Expression–Word Score (WE-Word)

Calculate the Written Expression–Word score (WE-Word) by dividing the number of words produced correctly by the total number of words. Start by circling any words that meet any of the following conditions:

- Words that are misspelled

- Words that have letters printed backward

- Words that are inflected wrong for the syntactic context (e.g., subject/verb agreement)

- Words that contain errors in word-level punctuation (i.e., word-level punctuation only, such as extra or a missing apostrophe—disregard sentence-level punctuation)

- Words that are repeated unnecessarily (e.g., "he got got out" but not for emphasis as in "really really big")

- Words that are missing and need to be inserted to make a sentence grammatically or semantically complete

The WE-Word score is a percentage score. To calculate it, you must first count the total number of words produced by the student. Then, subtract the number of error words from the total words to get the total words correct. Take the total words correct and divide by the total number of words. Finally, multiply the result by 100 to produce the WE-Word score. This student omitted one word in the sentence, "The children found him and put [him] back," but all other words were correct. The student produced 41 words for this story and made one word error.

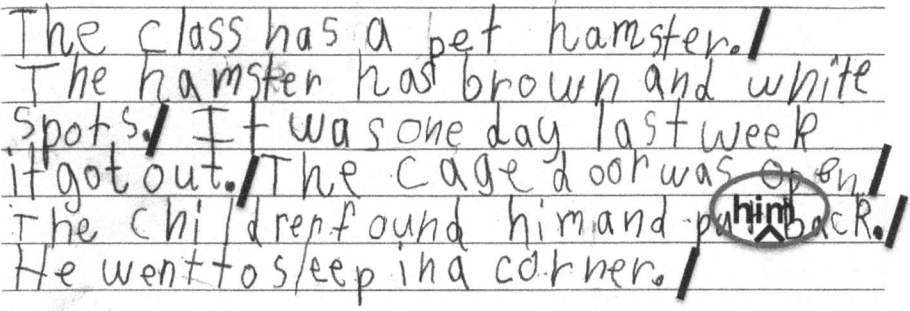

This student's Word score is calculated as follows:

$$\frac{41 \text{ total words} - 1 \text{ error word} = 40 \text{ correct words}}{41 \text{ total words}} \times 100 = 97.6\% \text{ (rounds to 98\%)}$$

The remainder of this section provides rules for counting words and word errors, followed by training in the grammatical skills and exercises for learning to divide T-units.

RULES FOR COUNTING WORDS AND WORD ERRORS

Counting Total Words

The following are rules for counting total words:

1. In any story, count a numeral (e.g., *2, 6, 15*) as a word.

2. In Story C, "When the School Closed," count "6 a.m." as two words no matter how the student spells, spaces, or punctuates the words. Examples are "six am" and "6 AM" (2 words each). "Six o'clock am" would count as 3 words.

3. In Story D, "The Building," count "grave yard" as one word even if the student puts a space in the middle (e.g., grave yard), which is how this compound word appears in the *Stimulus Book*.

4. Following are tips for achieving accuracy in counting total words:

   - Write subtotals every few lines and then add them up.

   - Count left to right and then drop down one row and count right to left to avoid skipping a line.

   - When counting to yourself, emphasize the number name (e.g., 10, 20) each time you complete a set of 10 and begin the next group of 10 (e.g., "eight, nine, TEN, eleven").

5. If a student clearly omits a word that is required to make the sentence grammatical, write it in, circle it, and count it as an error word, but do not add it to the total word count.

6. If the student includes a title or "the end," do not incorporate the words from those components in the total word count and do not include either element in the T-unit count.

Counting Error Words

Circle and count as error words any of the following:

1. Misspelled words, such as *sprised/surprised.* (If the same word is misspelled multiple times, be sure to circle and count each misspelled instance.)

2. Omitted words that would have to be added to make a sentence grammatical, such as "The hamster was out / [they] didn't know where to find it./"

3. Extra or substituted words, such as "The hamster *out* out." (The student probably intended to write "got out.")

4. Words that are not inflected correctly for the sentence, such as plural or tense endings missing or added, as in "The hamster *escape.*" Make a qualitative observation note if you think the inflectional error might reflect the student's oral language dialect, but still count it as an error word. The rationale for this decision is that there is no way to verify the source of variation. Students with language and literacy disorders are known to make changes in inflectional endings in their written language, and such discrepancies should not be undercounted for students who may come from diverse racial or ethnic backgrounds.

5. Words with a letter oriented in the wrong direction, such as *hab/had* or *qut/put.*

6. Words with inappropriate within-word punctuation, such as *wan't's/wants.*

7. If the student includes a title, do not count any error words that may appear in the title, but make a note about them under Qualitative Observations.

When Not to Count a Word as an Error

Do not count the following as "error words" because they are too difficult to count reliably:

1. Words with capitalization errors, such as *red Nose, sara, tHe,* or *monday*

2. Consistent handwriting issues, such as an *a* that looks like a *u* or failing to close the top of many letters

3. Sentence-level punctuation errors involving commas, missing periods, or question marks

WHAT IS A T-UNIT AND WHY DOES IT MATTER?

A T-unit is, "One main clause plus the subordinate clauses attached to or embedded within it" (Hunt, 1965, p. 49). That is, a T-unit is an independent clause with all of its dependent components so that it may stand alone as a fully complete grammatical unit. An independent clause must have a subject plus a verb, but it can have other components embedded in it or subordinated to it. An independent clause might begin with one of the coordinating conjunctions—*and, but, or, so.*

If T-units are like sentences, one could ask why not just mark off sentences to score the Written Expression (WE) subtest? The trouble with such an approach would be that examiners must all agree on where sentences begin and end. It would not work to use students' capitalization and end punctuation to make this decision because such skills have to be taught explicitly and they can vary widely across the school-age years. Examiners also need a rule for handling situations in which students string multiple clauses together with coordinating conjunctions to produce excessively long, run-on sentences. To avoid overcrediting run-on sentences, which potentially could be "interminable," Hunt (1965) defined *minimal terminable units* (T-units) as a main clause and its subordinated attached or embedded clauses. By doing so, he provided a consistent way to segment written language utterances on the basis of linguistic structure that could be used reliably by multiple examiners.

So, why does T-unit division matter? Consider the following two written examples:

1. The dog was big / and he went for a walk / but he chased a girl / and the girl screamed / so the boy pulled the leash. /

2. The big dog went for a walk and chased a girl, who screamed, which made the boy pull the leash. /

These two sentences convey essentially the same information, but are quite different in terms of their grammatical complexity. If we measure complexity as the number of words incorporated into a grammatical unit, it becomes apparent why T-units matter. If Example 1 were treated as a single sentence, it would have a length of 25 words, whereas Example 2 would have a length of 20 words and thus might be judged less complex. However, Example 1 actually consists of a string of 5 independent clauses (T-units) joined with coordinating conjunctions for a total of 25 words. If we use T-units as the unit of measure, Example 1 now averages 5.0 words per T-unit.

$$\frac{25 \text{ words}}{5 \text{ T-units}} = 5.0 \text{ words per T-unit}$$

On the other hand, Example 2 incorporates essentially the same information in a more complex single T-unit of 20 words.

$$\frac{20 \text{ words}}{1 \text{ T-unit}} = 20.0 \text{ words per T-unit}$$

Of course, syntactic measurements would never be based on such short samples, but these examples illustrate how T-unit division can make it possible to assign quantitative scores to grammatical units so they can be compared across samples in a meaningful way.

BRIEF REVIEW OF CLAUSE TYPES

Learning to divide language samples into T-units requires grammatical skills for identifying independent and dependent clauses. These clauses and subtypes are reviewed in this section.

Independent Clauses

A main clause (independent clause) is defined as a structure containing a subject (e.g., *Ben, Ben and Jerry*) and a verb phrase (e.g., *likes, like ice cream*). A main clause expresses a thought that can stand on its own, with no other words needed to express the main

Coordinating conjunctions
and
but
or
so

meaning. Two main clauses may be joined (coordinated) with one of the four coordinating conjunctions (*and, but, or, so*). In this case, each main clause joined with a coordinating conjunction expresses a thought that could stand on its own. Here are some examples:

*   The cage was open, / and the pet jumped out./ (2 T-units)

    [Two independent clauses in one sentence, joined by the coordinating conjunction *and*; Each independent clause is a separate T-unit.]

*   But it jumped out./ (1 T-unit)

    [One independent clause beginning with a coordinating conjunction, *but*]

*   The young children and the teacher saw the principal's daughter./ (1 T-unit)

    [One independent clause with a compound subject, *children* and *teacher*, but only one verb phrase]

*   The student has been writing./ (1 T-unit)

    [One independent clause with a single verb phrase with auxiliaries, *has been writing*]

Dependent Clauses

A dependent clause contains a subject and a verb but does not form a sentence that can stand alone. Instead, it adds to the meaning of the main clause. The three main types of dependent clauses function as adjectives, adverbs, and nouns. A T-unit that incorporates a dependent clause is considered complex because it combines two propositions (i.e., basic sentence meanings) into one sentence.

> Relative pronouns include
>
> who
> whose
> whom
> that
> which

A **relative (adjectival) clause** begins with a relative pronoun (e.g., *who, whose, whom, that, which*). It works like an adjective, providing information by modifying a noun or pronoun. Here are some examples:

*   They have a principal *whose daughter's name is Sara.* / (1 T-unit)

    [Relative (adjectival) clause modifying the direct object *principal*]

*   Sara, *who has a red nose,* is the principal's daughter./ (1 T-unit)

    [Relative (adjectival) clause modifying a subject noun phrase, *Sara*]

*   The red nose [*that*] *Sara had on* was scary./ (1 T-unit)

    [Relative (adjectival) clause modifying a subject noun phrase (*the red nose*), with optional relative pronoun (*that*)]

> Relative pronouns often signal the presence of a dependent clause.

A **subordinate (adverbial) clause** begins with a subordinate conjunction (e.g., *after, when, because, so that*) and works like an adverb, providing information about temporal, locational, causal, or other relationships. Here are some examples:

*   Some of the children cried *after they saw her.* / (1 T-unit)

    [Italics show an independent clause with a subordinate (adverbial) clause at the end of the T-unit.]

- *Because the hamster escaped,* the class was upset. / (1 T-unit)

  [Italics show a subordinate (adverbial) clause at the beginning of the T-unit.]

A **nominal (noun) clause** functions like a noun. Nominalization can occur at the beginning of the sentence, functioning as the subject, or at the end, functioning as the object (complement) of the main verb. A nominal clause may be introduced by indefinite pronouns such as *what, that,* and *who.* Following are some examples:

Subordinate conjunctions include
although
as soon as
if
since
so that
until
when
whether
while

- *That the hamster escaped* was a big problem. / (1 T-unit)

  [Italics show a dependent (nominal) clause functioning as the subject of the sentence.]

- She saw *that the hamster escaped.* / (1 T-unit)

  [Italics show a dependent (nominal) clause functioning as the object (complement) of the sentence.]

Nominal clauses operate as the subject or object of a sentence.

- The children hoped [*that*] *they would find the hamster.* / (1 T-unit)

  [Italics show a dependent (noun) clause functioning as the object complement of the sentence.]

- I know *who left the door open.* / (1 T-unit)

  [A dependent (noun) clause functioning as the object complement of the sentence.]

TIPS FOR MARKING T-UNITS IN TILLS WRITTEN EXPRESSION (WE) SAMPLES

The T-unit is based on linguistic units. Ignore children's punctuation when dividing T-units. Some conjunctions are tricky.

- *So* is a coordinating conjunction (often used to start sentences), but *so* also can function as a subordinate conjunction when it takes the meaning of *so that.*

  Example: The children couldn't find the hamster, / *so* they didn't know what to do. / (2 T-units)

  Example: The children looked for the hamster *so* they could put it back in the cage. / (1 T-unit)

- *But* is a coordinating conjunction (often used to start a new T-unit).

  Example: The children looked for the hamster / *but* they couldn't find it. / (2 T-units)

  Example: The children looked for the hamster but couldn't find it (1 T-unit because the subject of the second clause has been removed)

- *Because* is a subordinating conjunction that introduces an adverbial clause (subordinated to a main clause). Therefore, *because* is part of the main clause T-unit.

  Example: The children were sad *because* they couldn't find the hamster. / (1 T-unit)

- Count fragments created because of missing words as separate T-units.

   Example: The hamster was out / didn't know where to find it / (2 T-units; the second subject [They] is missing, which would count as an error word)

Some adverbial clauses are harder to recognize because they have nonfinite forms of verbs and do not have a subordinate conjunction at the beginning. Consider the example *"Seeing that she had a fever,* her mother kept her home from school." In this sentence, the verb *seeing* is a nonfinite verb, meaning that it is not marked for tense or number (the *-ing* inflection is a progressive aspect marker, not tense). Infinitive forms of verbs are also nonfinite, as in "The doctor prescribed antibiotics *to halt the bacterial infection."* This is an adverbial clause of purpose (where "in order" could be inserted before the "to"), which is quite common. All verbs in main clauses, as well as most verbs in dependent clauses, are finite, meaning that they are marked for tense and number.

Practice Identifying T-Units

Consider the examples in the chart on the next page to help you to check your understanding of the rules reviewed in this section. To use the chart to reinforce your learning, cover the columns showing the number of T-units and explanation with a piece of paper or cardstock so that the answers and explanations are not visible until you try to answer each one.

TRAINING EXAMPLES AND PRACTICE EXERCISES

The following section includes training examples for a variety of the components you will need to score when you administer the Written Expression (WE) subtest. Each training example gives you a set of sentences followed by steps you should take to score the examples. An answer key is provided for each training example following all the training examples. After these training examples, you will then find a set of practice exercises to help you reinforce your knowledge.

Phrases and Clauses Training Example

Read the five phrases and clauses in the box below, and then take the actions in the bulleted list that follows, marking directly on the five examples in the box.

---

1. The girl who was the principal's daughter put on the wig before she came in the class.

2. That the children cried made Sara feel bad.

3. The skunk that was very hungry took the cookies after he ran away.

4. The janitor searched because the skunks that ate the cookies were hiding in the cafeteria.

5. Because the children who were taking care of it left the cage door open, the hamster escaped.

- Circle the verb (or verb phrase) of each main clause (just the verb, not its object).

- Single underline the subject(s) of the main clause.

- Double underline any subordinate (adverbial) clauses.

- Put any relative (adjectival) clauses in parentheses.

- Put any nominal clauses in square brackets.

Practice identifying T-units: Cover the number of T-units and explanation columns to check your knowledge as you read down the list of examples at the left.

	Number of T-units	Explanation
The class has a pet of a hamster.	1	The presence of one subject + predicate indicates one main clause. Note that the grammatical error is ignored in determining the T-unit.
The hamster has brown and white spots.	1	Despite the conjunction "and," there is only one main clause.
The hamter got got up and got out.	1	There are two verbs here (a compound verb phrase) but only one subject, making this one main clause. Note that the spelling error and word repetition are ignored in determining the T-units.
The Principal's Daughter (title written out by the student)	N/A	Titles are excluded from T-unit calculations.
She had on makeup and a wig.	1	The conjunction "and" forms a complex object phrase, but there is only one main clause because there is only one subject ("She").
A ball, a red one, was on her nose.	1	One subject ("A ball") and one verb ("was") form one main clause.
Some childrens crited and they were scared.	2	The coordinating conjunction ("and") joins two separate ideas that each contain a subject and a verb. Main clause 1: "Some children crited" Main clause 2: "they were scared" Note that the spelling error is ignored in determining the T-units.
then she took off her wig so the children were happy because they new Sara	2	The coordinating conjunction "so" separates two main clauses: Main clause 1: "then she took off her wig" Main clause 2: "the children were happy" The subordinating conjunction "because" indicates "because they new Sara" is a dependent clause that tells why the children were happy. Note that the capitalization and spelling errors are ignored in determining the T-units.
Our school was closed last Wednesday, despite being a school day.	1	The clause "despite being a school day" cannot stand alone, making it a dependent clause.
He smelled something strong that almost knowcked him over and it was a skunk	2	The coordinating conjunction "and" joins two main clauses: Main clause 1: "He smelled something strong" Main clause 2: "It was a skunk" The clause "that almost knowcked him over" is a relative clause.
He looked in the library and the cafeteria before he found the skunks.	1	The conjunction "and" in this case separates two object phrases ("the library" and "the cafeteria") rather than two complete subject + predicate units. The conjunction "before" is a subordinate conjunction. The clause "before he found the skunks" describes when he looked (the main verb). Therefore, it is an adverbial clause.
There were two eating cookies.	1	"Eating cookies" cannot stand on its own apart from "There were two," making it a dependent clause.
People talked about its history, which some people knew.	1	"Which some people knew" modifies "its history," making it a dependent clause.
The building, that was a hospital, was used in a war long ago.	1	"That was a hospital" is a relative clause.
They did not care but then something happened.	2	The coordinating conjunction "but" joins two complete subject + predicate clauses. Main clause 1: "They did not care" Main clause 2: "then something happened."
They raised money and saved the building.	1	The omission of a second subject after the conjunction "and" indicates that this is one main clause.
They saved something else more important to them.	1	"They saved something else" is the main clause. "More important to them" modifies "something else," making it a dependent clause.

Answer Key for Training Examples: Phrases and Clauses

1. <u>The girl</u> (who was the principal's daughter) (put on) the wig <u>before she came in the class</u>.

2. [That the children cried] (made) Sara feel bad.

3. <u>The skunk</u> (that was very hungry) (took) the cookies <u>after he ran away</u>.

4. <u>The janitor</u> (searched) <u>because the skunks (that ate the cookies) were hiding in the cafeteria</u>.

5. <u>Because the children (who were taking care of it) left the cage door open</u>, the hamster (escaped).

Note: All of these examples are 1 T-unit in length.

T-Unit Division Training Examples

Based on the information provided earlier in this Section IIIA, determine which of the following examples is one T-unit and which needs to be divided into more than one T-unit. Place a slash mark (/) after each T-unit in the examples in the box below. After working on the following 14 examples, check your T-units marks with the Answer Key that follows to make sure you understand explanations of T-unit divisions.

---

1. She shut the cage door so the hamster wouldn't get out.

2. She always wanted to be a clown so she came on Monday.

3. They looked for the hamster, but they didn't find him because he was hiding in the corner.

4. They knew that it was a hospital and that it was used in a war.

5. The hamster was in the cage. Then, something happened!

6. Then they let them go in the deep, dark woods. Bye-bye skunks!

7. They put him in his cage and fell asleep.

8. He got got of his cage and the door was open.

9. They were eating cookies. O boy were they hungry.

10. When she took off her red nose the children were happy . . . After they saw it was Sara.

11. The children looked for him and found him and put him back in his cage. So he found a corner and went to sleep.

12. The children was spris to see him.

13. She wan't's to put on a clown sut she came Monday at school

14. They made something else which was their progress. That was the key.

Answer Key for T-Unit Identification

1. She shut the cage door so the hamster wouldn't get out. / (1 T-unit)

   So has the meaning of *so that,* making the clause that follows subordinate: one independent and one dependent clause. Because there is only one independent clause, this is 1 T-unit.

2. She always wanted to be a clown / so she came on Monday. / (2 T-units)

   So in this example is a coordinating conjunction connecting two independent clauses.

3. They looked for the hamster, / but they didn't find him because he was hiding in the corner. / (2 T-units)

   But in this example is a coordinating conjunction connecting two independent clauses.

   Because is a subordinating conjunction, introducing a dependent (adverbial) clause, so it is *not* marked off as a new T-unit.

4. They knew that it was a hospital and that it was used in a war. / (1 T-unit)

   This sentence contains two object complement (nominal) clauses that are themselves coordinated with *and.* The first is *that it was a hospital,* and the second is *that it was used in a war.* Both dependent clauses are "governed" by the verb *knew* in the main clause. Therefore, this is 1 T-unit.

5. The hamster was in the cage. / Then, something happened! / (2 T-units)

   Then is a starter (often written as "and then"). It functions much like a coordinating conjunction in this instance and begins a new T-unit.

6. Then they let them go in the deep, dark woods. / Bye-bye skunks! / (2 T-units)

   Fragments or short utterances are treated as separate T-units (sometimes called C-units) if they can stand alone in conversational speech.

7. They put him in his cage / and [he] fell asleep. / (2 T-units; 1 error word)

   This sentence has an omitted subject (*he*); *they* did not fall asleep; T-units are not affected by grammatical errors; fragments are counted as separate T-units to avoid overcrediting the child's grammatical development; the missing "he" would be counted as a word error. The way this is written, "they" [the children] would be the subject of both verb phrases, and that changes the meaning of the story and is likely not the student's intended meaning.

8. He got <u>got</u> of his cage / and the door was open. / (2 T-units; 1 error word)

   This sentence has an extra verb, *got,* and is missing the word *out.* T-units are not affected by grammar or spelling errors.

9. They were eating cookies. / O boy were they hungry. / (2 T-units)

   Oh boy is an interjection and considered part of the following T-unit.

10. When she took off her red nose the children were happy . . . After they saw it was Sara. / (1 T-unit)

    After they saw it was Sara is a subordinate clause, which is considered part of the T-unit, even though it is punctuated separately. T-units are not affected by the student's punctuation.

11. The children looked for him and found him and put him back in his cage. / So he found a corner and went to sleep. / (2 T-units)

Compound verb phrases are part of a single T-unit if they have the same subject.

12. The children <u>was</u> <u>spris</u> to see him. / (1 T-unit; 2 error words)

T-units are not affected by spelling and verb tense errors, *spris* for *surprised*. The nonfinite verb phrase (*to see him*) is a noncomplementing infinitive.

13. She <u>wan't's</u> to put on a clown <u>sut</u> / she came Monday <u>at</u> school / (2 T-units; 3 error words)

T-units are not affected by incorrect punctuation, *wan't's* for *wants*.

T-units are not affected by incorrect grammar, *at* for *to*.

The words "wan't's" and "at" would be circled and counted as word errors, along with *sut/suit*.

14. They made something else which was their progress. / That was the key. / (2 T-units)

That is a pronoun functioning as the subject of a new independent clause. *Which* is a relative pronoun beginning a relative clause.

Practice Exercises

Following are 13 exercises to help you practice your skills in scoring the Written Expression (WE) subtest. Follow the five instructions below. An answer key is provided for each exercise after all of the exercises. In all of the practice exercises, spelling and punctuation are maintained as produced in the children's original hand-written stories. Ignore the students' punctuation when marking T-units.

1. Mark a slash at the end of each T-unit.

2. Underline or circle any word that should be counted as a word error. Word errors include misspelling errors, within-word punctuation errors, any word or cluster of omitted words (you can show omitted words/morphemes with *word or *morpheme), and any word that must be modified to make the sentence grammatical. Note that each omission error counts as one error word even if it would take two replacement words to make the sentence grammatically correct.

3. Count the total words and enter the total at the end of each practice exercise.

4. After completing each practice set, compare your responses to the corresponding key and seek to understand the rationale for any discrepancies by returning to the training examples in this section or the *Examiner's Manual*.

5. Complete additional practice exercises as needed.

Practice Exercise 1

> There was an old building. People think that it might have been used for the Civil War. This building was a hospital where many people died. Behind this building there was a grave yard. It was hidden. People wanted to sell the land and tear it down. The people of the city saved it because it was there history.
>
> Total T-units: __   Total error words: __   Total words: __

Practice Exercise 2

Last Wednesday, a school day, our school was closed all day. The janitor came at six o'clock in the morning and opened the school, but he smelt a strong skunk smell that almost made him pass out. He opened the doors and left them open as he searched. He found two, hungry, skunks eating in the cafeteria. He called the animal control department right away. The workers came took the skunks and let them go in the woods.

Total T-units: __   Total error words: __   Total words: __

Practice Exercise 3

There was a building. It was old. People talked about it. It was used in a war. It was the Civil War. Many soldiers died. There were buried. People did not think about it. They did not care. Then something happen. They wanted to sell the land. They wrote articles. They gave speeches They raised money. They saved the graveyard. They saved something else. It was their history. that was more important.

Total T-units: __   Total error words: __   Total words: __

Practice Exercise 4

The class got a pet it is a hamster it got out the cage the cage was open the Door was open the children found it we put hime Back in the cage he found a corner he whent to sleep.

Total T-units: __   Total error words: __   Total words: __

Practice Exercise 5

Last Wednesday our school was closed all day on a school day. When the janitor came at six o'clock am to open the school, he smelled something. The smell was strong and it was coming from a skunk. He had almost fell over because of the skunk. He started searching in the cafeteria, opened the doors and left them open. The janitor had found two very hungry skunks snacking on cookies. Right away he called the animal control department. When the workers came and took the two skunks and let them go in the woods.

Total T-units: __   Total error words: __   Total words: __

Practice Exercise 6

Our school was closed last Wednesday it was a school day it was closed all day a janitor came at six o'clock am and opened the school and smelled something strong it was a skunk it almost nocked him over he open all the doors He searched all over and found 2 skunks in the cafeteria They were eating cookies they were very hungry he call the animal control department right away and the workers came and took the skunks and let them go in the woods.

Total T-units: __   Total error words: __   Total words: __

Practice Exercise 7

There was an old building that was used during the civil war as a hospital. Many of the soldiers died and were burried in the graveyard behind the building. People didn't think about the building because it was hidden and they didn't care about it. Then the city wanted to tear it down to sell the land and suddenly the people started to care. They decided to write articles, and give speeches, as well as raise money. After all their hard work they were able to save the building and the graveyard. But most importantly they saved their history.

Total T-units: __   Total error words: __   Total words: __

Practice Exercise 8

A school was closed on Wednesday it was school time today it whey six o'clock a.m. they so a skunk and they whint to go eat cookies and they wher still hungry and they whint to the woods.

Total T-units: __   Total error words: __   Total words: __

Practice Exercise 9

It was Wednesday I walk to school. The school was closed because two skunks were in the school. The janitor called the animal control department. They catch the skunks and put them in the woods.

Total T-units: __   Total error words: __   Total words: __

Practice Exercise 10

Our school was closed last Wednesday on a schoool and it was closed all day then the janitor came at six o'clock a.m, and open the school then he smelled something strong it was a skunk that almost knocked him over. He open the doors left them open then he searched. He looked in the cafeteria and found two skunks that were eating cookies and very hungry. Then called the animal control department right aaway then the worker came took the skunks let them go in the woods

Total T-units: __   Total error words: __   Total words: __

Practice Exercise 11

There was an old building that was a hospital during the Civil War, and because there were no records no one knew how old it was. Many soldiers who had died were buried in the graveyard that was almost hidden behind the building. People didn't think or care about it until the city wanted to tear the old hospital building down and sell the land. The people were suddenly writing speeches and raising money. They saved the building and graveyard but more importantly they saved their history.

Total T-units: __   Total error words: __   Total words: __

Practice Exercise 12

There was an old building, but nobody knew how old it really was. There weren't any records of the building of how old it was, but they only knew two things about the building. They knew that it was a hospital and that it was used in a war. The war that it was used in was the Civil War. And in that hospital many soldiers had died. The dead soldiers were buried in the graveyard behind the hospital. The graveyard is still there. People didn't think about the graveyard behind the building. Cause the graveyard was almost hidden. They didn't care about the building. Then, something happened! The city wanted to tear down the building. The city wanted to sell the land. People suddenly cared about the old hospital building

Total T-units: __   Total error words: __   Total words: __

Practice Exercise 13

THe class Haves a pet. it is a Hamst but it got out of tHe cage. THe class now tHe door cage THey noiw tHat tHey lock tHe cage. THe cHildren found Him in the conren of the wall sleeping.

Total T-units: __   Total error words: __   Total words: __

Answer Key for Practice Exercise 1

There was an old building. / People think that it might have been used for the Civil War. / This building was a hospital where many people died. / Behind this building there was a grave yard. / It was hidden. / People wanted to sell the land and tear it down. / The people of the city saved it because it was <u>there</u> history. /

Total T-units: <u>7</u>   Total error words: <u>1</u> (there/their)
Total words: <u>58</u> (grave yard counts as 1 word)

Answer Key for Practice Exercise 2

Last Wednesday, a school day, our school was closed all day. / The janitor came at six o'clock in the morning and opened the school, / but he <u>smelt</u> a strong skunk smell that almost made him pass out. / He opened the doors and left them open as he searched. / He found two, hungry, skunks eating in the cafeteria. / He called the animal control department right away. / The workers came took the skunks and let them go in the woods. /

Total T-units: <u>7</u>   Total error words: <u>1</u> (smelt/smelled)   Total words: <u>78</u>

Answer Key for Practice Exercise 3

There was a building. / It was old. / People talked about it. / It was used in a war. / It was the Civil War. / Many soldiers died. / <u>There</u> were buried. / People did not think about it. / They did not care. / Then something <u>happen*ed</u>. / They wanted to sell the land. / They wrote articles. / They gave speeches / They raised money. / They saved the graveyard. / They saved something else. / It was their history. / that was more important. /

Total T-units: <u>18</u>   Total error words: <u>2</u> (there/they, happen/happened)
Total words: <u>72</u>

Answer Key for Practice Exercise 4

The class got a pet / it is a hamster / it got out *of the cage / the cage was open / the Door was open / the children found it / we put hime Back in the cage / he found a corner / he whent to sleep. /

Total T-units: 9 Total error words: 3 ("of" was omitted, hime/him, whent/went)
Total words: 41

(Don't count omitted words in the total, but do count them as error words.)

Answer Key for Practice Exercise 5

Last Wednesday our school was closed all day on a school day. / When the janitor came at six o'clock am to open the school, he smelled something. / The smell was strong / and it was coming from a skunk. / He had almost fell over because of the skunk. / He started searching in the cafeteria, opened the doors and left them open. / The janitor had found two very hungry skunks snacking on cookies. / Right away he called the animal control department. / When the workers came and *they [and/*they count as 1 error word] took the two skunks and let them go in the woods. /

Total T-units: 9 Total error words: 2 (fell/fallen and/and they) Total words: 95

Note: It is not the best parallel structure to write "He started searching in the cafeteria, opened the doors and left them open," but this is not about correcting students' sentence structure to improve the literary quality. Rather, the rule of thumb is to ask, "Can you say that?" Therefore, no changes are made in this construction and it is counted as 1 T-unit. The last sentence would be incomplete, however, if "and" were not changed to "they." This sentence should read, "When the workers came they took the two skunks and let them go in the woods."

Answer Key for Practice Exercise 6

Our school was closed last Wednesday /it was a school day / it was closed all day / a janitor came at six o'clock am and opened the school and smelled something strong / it was a skunk / it almost nocked him over / he open*ed all the doors / He searched all over and found 2 skunks in the cafeteria / They were eating cookies / they were very hungry / he call*ed the animal control department right away / and the workers came and took the skunks and let them go in the woods. /

Total T-units: 12 Total error words: 3 (nocked/knocked, open/opened, call/called)
Total words: 87

Note: Standard edited American English is used in scoring the WE subtest, but it is important to be aware of possible dialectal influences of the student's oral language on his or her written language. If the student who wrote this sample were a speaker of African American English, the student's spoken dialect could have influenced the omission of the past tense markers on "open" and "call"; however, students with language impairment often demonstrate a pattern of omitting verb inflections. Therefore, these two omissions are counted as errors. If you suspect that dialect difference might account for a student having a low WE-Word score, you should note this under Qualitative Observations and avoid using the WE-Word score in making decisions about whether the student has a language disorder.

Answer Key for Practice Exercise 7

There was an old building that was used during the civil war as a hospital. / Many of the soldiers died and were <u>burried</u> in the graveyard behind the building. / People didn't think about the building because it was hidden / and they didn't care about it. / Then the city wanted to tear it down to sell the land / and suddenly the people started to care. / They decided to write articles, and give speeches, as well as raise money. / After all their hard work they were able to save the building and the graveyard. / But most importantly they saved their history. /

Total T-units: <u>9</u>   Total error words: <u>1</u> (burried/buried)   Total words: <u>99</u>

Answer Key for Practice Exercise 8

A school was closed on Wednesday / it was school time today / it <u>whey</u> six o'clock a.m. / they <u>so</u> a skunk / and they <u>whint</u> to go eat cookies / and they <u>wher</u> still hungry / and they <u>whint</u> to the woods. /

Total T-units: <u>7</u>   Total error words: <u>5</u> (whey/when, so/saw, whint/went, wher/were, whint/went)   Total words: <u>38</u>

Note: You could make a Qualitative Observation about "they" being used with unclear referents, but these usages do not count as word errors.

Answer Key for Practice Exercise 9

It was Wednesday / I <u>walk*ed</u> to school. / The school was closed because two skunks were in the school. / The janitor called the animal control department. / They <u>catch</u> the skunks and put them in the woods. /

Total T-units: <u>5</u>   Total error words: <u>2</u> (walk/walked, catch/caught)   Total words: <u>35</u>

Answer Key for Practice Exercise 10

Our school was closed last Wednesday on a <u>schoool</u> <u>*day</u> / and it was closed all day / then the janitor came at six o'clock a.m, and <u>open*ed</u> the school / then he smelled something strong / it was a skunk that almost knocked him over. / He <u>open*ed</u> the doors <u>*and</u> left them open / then he searched. / He looked in the cafeteria and found two skunks that were eating cookies and very hungry. / Then <u>*he</u> called the animal control department right <u>aaway</u> / then the worker came took the skunks <u>*and</u> let them go in the woods /

Total T-units: <u>10</u>   Total error words: <u>8</u> (schoool/school, *day was missing, open/opened, open/opened, *and was missing, *he was missing, aaway/away, *and was missing)   Total words: <u>88</u>

Answer Key for Practice Exercise 11

There was an old building that was a hospital during the Civil War, / and because there were no records no one knew how old it was. / Many soldiers who had died were buried in the graveyard that was almost hidden behind the building. / People didn't think or care about it until the city wanted to tear the old hospital building down and sell the land. / The people were suddenly writing speeches and raising money. / They saved the building and graveyard / but more importantly they saved their history. /

Total T-units: <u>7</u>   Total error words: <u>0</u>   Total words: <u>87</u>

Answer Key for Practice Exercise 12

There was an old building, / but nobody knew how old it really was. / There weren't any records of the building of how old it was, / but they only knew two things about the building. / They knew that it was a hospital and that it was used in a war. / The war that it was used in was the Civil War. / And in that hospital many soldiers had died. / The dead soldiers were buried in the graveyard behind the hospital. / The graveyard is still there. / People didn't think about the graveyard behind the building. Cause the graveyard was almost hidden. / They didn't care about the building. / Then, something happened! / The city wanted to tear down the building. / The city wanted to sell the land. / People suddenly cared about the old hospital building /

Total T-units: 15   Total error words: 1 (cause/because)   Total words: 131

Note: This sample provides an example of why it is unwise to use the student's punctuation to divide T-units. In this case, the student inserted a period in the sentence, "People didn't think about the graveyard behind the building. Cause the graveyard was almost hidden." Nevertheless, this construction is 1 T-unit.

Answer Key for Practice Exercise 13

THe class Haves a pet. / it is a Hamst / but it got out of tHe cage. / THe class now tHe door cage *was_locked / THey noiw tHat tHey lock*ed tHe cage. / THe cHildren found Him in the conren of the wall sleeping. /

Total T-units: 6   Total error words: 7 (haves/have, hamst/hamster, now/knew, *was_open omitted phrase, noiw/knew, lock/locked, conren/corner)   Total words: 40

Note: The words "was open" were needed to complete the fourth T-unit, "The class [knew] the cage door [was locked]." These two omitted words count as one error word, however, and they are not included in the total word count.

REFERENCES

DeMaagd-Slager, M.N. (2011). *Learning to divide discourse into minimal terminable units (T-units): Reliability after brief instruction* (Unpublished master's thesis). Kalamazoo: Western Michigan University.

Hunt, K.W. (1965). *Grammatical structures written at three grade levels.* Urbana, IL: National Council of Teachers of English.

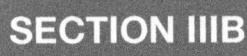

Additional Scored Examples for the Written Expression Subtest

This section provides additional examples of Written Expression (WE) samples for Stories A, B, C, and D, which have been scored for you. These stories were selected to illustrate some of the challenging decisions that must be made when scoring the WE subtest.

EXAMPLE 1

This example was written by a girl (age 7;1) with language literacy risks.

> The class Pet ~~was~~ it the class // it was a hamster // it got lost in the week, one day // the hamster had brown and white (spots) // He (wit) to (sleep) // the gate was open // and he got lost (it) the school they (poot) (he) back in the cage // and the (childre) (woet) out the door and found the (hamer) out the door //

WRITTEN EXPRESSION CONTENT UNITS SCORING FORM					
Story A: "The Class Pet" (p. 69)					
1. The <u>class</u> has a <u>pet</u>.	0	(1)	9. The <u>door</u> was open.	0	(1)
2. It is a <u>hamster</u>.	0	(1)	10. The children <u>looked</u>.	(0)	1
3. The hamster has <u>spots</u>.	(0)	1	11. The children <u>found</u> him.	0	(1)
4. Some are <u>brown</u>.	0	(1)	12. They <u>put him back</u>.	0	(1)
5. Some are <u>white</u>.	0	(1)	13. They put him in the <u>cage</u>.	0	(1)
6. It <u>got out</u>.	0	(1)	14. They closed the <u>door</u>.	0	(1)
7. It was one day <u>last week</u>.	0	(1)	15. He found a <u>corner</u>.	(0)	1
8. The cage was <u>open</u>.	0	(1)	16. He went to <u>sleep</u>.	0	(1)
				Content Units total	13 /16

6;6–7

Discourse Score	<u>13</u> Content Units / 16 possible × 100 = <u>81</u> % Content Included
Sentence Score	<u>13</u> Content Units / <u>9</u> T-units* = <u>1.44</u> Sentence Score (record 2 decimal places)
Word Score	<u>60</u> Total Words − <u>10</u> Error Words = <u>50</u> Total Correct Words / <u>60</u> Total Words × 100 = <u>83</u> % Words Correct

EXAMPLE 2

This example was written by a girl (age 8;3) with language learning disability.

The class has a pet It is a hamster
The hamster has spots
Some are brown
It got out Too cage door children (put him) (The)
back corner sleep
(He) (Found) (a)
(he) (went) (to)

6:6–7

WRITTEN EXPRESSION CONTENT UNITS SCORING FORM
Story A: "The Class Pet" (p. 69)

1. The class has a pet.	0	(1)	9. The door was open.	0	(1)
2. It is a hamster.	0	(1)	10. The children looked.	(0)	1
3. The hamster has spots.	0	(1)	11. The children found him.	(0)	1
4. Some are brown.	0	(1)	12. They put him back.	0	(1)
5. Some are white.	(0)	1	13. They put him in the cage.	(0)	1
6. It got out.	0	(1)	14. They closed the door.	(0)	1
7. It was one day last week.	(0)	1	15. He found a corner.	0	(1)
8. The cage was open.	(0)	1	16. He went to sleep.	0	(1)
				Content Units total	9 /16

Discourse Score	__9__ Content Units / 16 possible × 100 = __56__% Content Included
Sentence Score	__9__ Content Units / __9__ T-units* = __1.0__ Sentence Score (record 2 decimal places)
Word Score	__26__ Total Words − __13__ Error Words = __13__ Total Correct Words / __26__ Total Words × 100 = __50__% Words Correct

EXAMPLE 3

This example was written by a girl (age 7;0) with normal language. Note the missing word on Line 4, "are," which would be required to make the sentence grammatical. The rule of thumb for counting missing words is to add the minimal possible to make a sentence grammatical.

The class has a pet./
It is a hamster./
The hamster has spots./
Some (are) brown/some are white./
It got out./
It was one day last week/
The cage was open/so was The Door/
The (cids) looked for (hem)/They found (him)
They put him back in his cage/
They closed the door/
He went to The corner/ He went to sleep/

6;6–7

WRITTEN EXPRESSION CONTENT UNITS SCORING FORM						
Story A: "The Class Pet" (p. 69)						
1. The class has a pet.	0	①	9. The door was open.	0	①	
2. It is a hamster.	0	①	10. The children looked.	0	①	
3. The hamster has spots.	0	①	11. The children found him.	0	①	
4. Some are brown.	0	①	12. They put him back.	0	①	
5. Some are white.	0	①	13. They put him in the cage.	0	①	
6. It got out.	0	①	14. They closed the door.	0	①	
7. It was one day last week.	0	①	15. He found a corner.	0	①	
8. The cage was open.	0	①	16. He went to sleep.	0	①	
				Content Units total	16	/16

Discourse Score	__16__ Content Units / 16 possible × 100 = __100__ % Content Included
Sentence Score	__16__ Content Units / __15__ T-units* = __1.07__ Sentence Score (record 2 decimal places)
Word Score	__62__ Total Words − __4__ Error Words = __58__ Total Correct Words / __62__ Total Words × 100 = __93__ % Words Correct

EXAMPLE 4

This example was written by a boy (age 10;0) with language learning disability. It provides an example of a student changing the meaning of a content unit. Instead of writing that "Sara came Monday to our school with makeup and wig on," the student wrote, "Sara came Monday to our school with no makeup or wig." This phrase was treated as one error word for scoring purposes. The student may have meant "on" rather than "no" or may have misread the original content unit. Using the word "no" made the word "or" fit the context, so it was not counted as an error word. Note that the two word errors in the top line are due to missing apostrophes prior to the possessive morphemes.

8–10	WRITTEN EXPRESSION CONTENT UNITS SCORING FORM					
	Story B: "The Principal's Daughter" (p. 71)					
1. We have a principal.	0	(1)	11. It was big.	0	(1)	
2. The principal has a daughter.	0	(1)	12. She looked scary.	0	(1)	
3. Her name is Sara.	0	(1)	13. She walked into a class.	0	(1)	
4. She wants to be a clown.	0	(1)	14. The children were young.	0	(1)	
5. She came Monday.	0	(1)	15. The children saw her.	0	(1)	
6. She came to our school.	0	(1)	16. Some children cried.	0	(1)	
7. She had on makeup.	(0)	1	17. They were scared.	0	(1)	
8. She had on a wig.*	(0)	1	18. She took off her wig.	0	(1)	
9. A ball was on her nose.	0	(1)	19. The children were happy.	0	(1)	
10. It was red.	0	(1)	20. They knew Sara.	0	(1)	
			Content Units total			18 /20

*Note: If child writes "dress" or "attire," score 1 for wig but 0 for makeup or ball on nose.

Discourse Score	18 Content Units / 20 possible × 100 = 90 % Content Included
Sentence Score	18 Content Units / 11 T-units* = 1.64 Sentence Score (record 2 decimal places)
Word Score	65 Total Words – 4 Error Words = 61 Total Correct Words / 65 Total Words × 100 = 94 % Words Correct

*Note: For more information about how to calculate T-units, see pages 74–77 in the Examiner's Manual.
Qualitative observations:

EXAMPLE 5

This example was written by a girl (age 9;3) with language learning disability. It provides an example of what to do with words that do not make sense or fit the context ("inside"): Treat them as error words. Error words include "principal" and "daughter" on Line 2, which are missing the apostrophe plus *s* possessive morpheme endings.

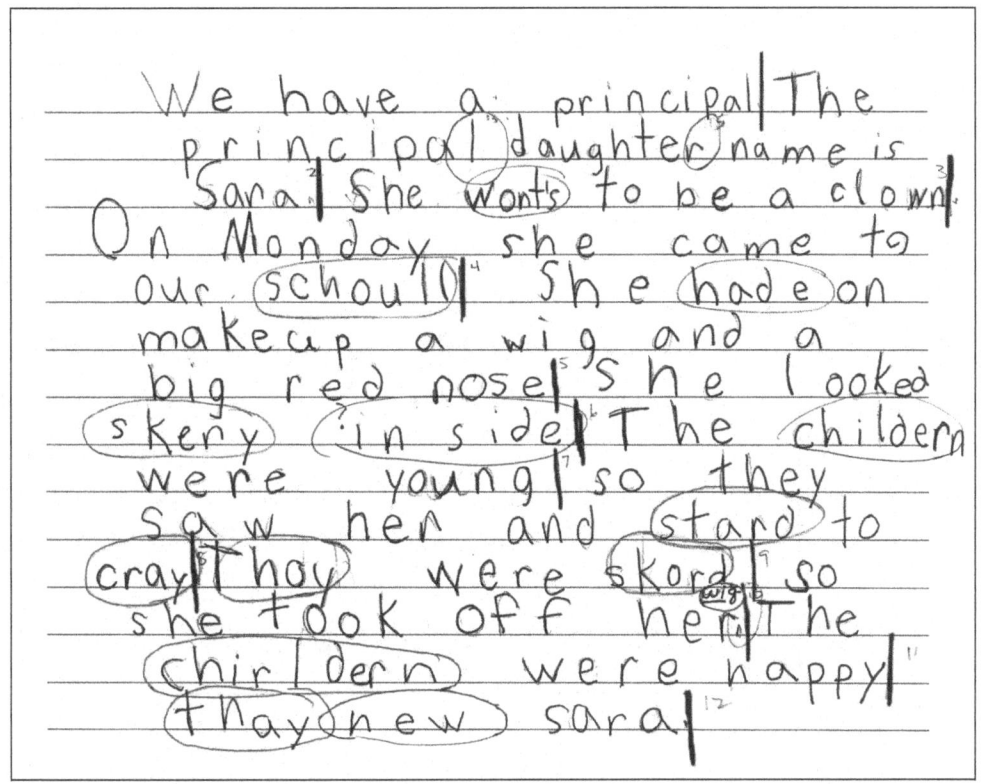

8–10

WRITTEN EXPRESSION CONTENT UNITS SCORING FORM					
Story B: "The Principal's Daughter" (p. 71)					
1. We have a <u>principal</u>.	0	(1)	11. It was <u>big</u>.	0	(1)
2. The principal has a <u>daughter</u>.	0	(1)	12. She looked <u>scary</u>.	0	(1)
3. Her <u>name</u> is <u>Sara</u>.	0	(1)	13. She walked into a <u>class</u>.	(0)	1
4. She wants to be a <u>clown</u>.	0	(1)	14. The children were <u>young</u>.	0	(1)
5. She came <u>Monday</u>.	0	(1)	15. The children <u>saw</u> her.	0	(1)
6. She came to our <u>school</u>.	0	(1)	16. Some children <u>cried</u>.	0	(1)
7. She had on <u>makeup</u>.	0	(1)	17. They were <u>scared</u>.	0	(1)
8. She had on a <u>wig</u>.*	0	(1)	18. She <u>took off</u> her <u>wig</u>.	(0)	1
9. A <u>ball</u> was on her <u>nose</u>.	(0)	1	19. The children were <u>happy</u>.	0	(1)
10. It was <u>red</u>.	0	(1)	20. They <u>knew Sara</u>.	0	(1)
				Content Units total	17 /20

*Note: If child writes "dress" or "attire," score 1 for wig but 0 for makeup or ball on nose.

Discourse Score	17 Content Units / 20 possible × 100 = 85 % Content Included
Sentence Score	17 Content Units / 12 T-units* = 1.42 Sentence Score (record 2 decimal places)
Word Score	65 Total Words − 16 Error Words = 49 Total Correct Words / 65 Total Words × 100 = 75 % Words Correct

*Note: For more information about how to calculate T-units, see pages 74–77 in the *Examiner's Manual*.
Qualitative observations:

EXAMPLE 6

This example was written by a boy (13;3) with normal language. Note the T-unit fragment "When he smelled a strong smell that almost knocked him over." This is a subordinate clause with an embedded relative clause. Because it is not connected logically to an independent clause, it is marked as a separate T-unit so as not to inflate the sentence score. The phrase "a lot" counts as two words no matter whether the student spaces the words that way or not.

Last (Wednsday) our school was closed all day! Our janitor came in at 6 a.m. when he smelled a strong smell that almost knocked him over.* It was a skunk! He left the doors open while he searched the library and cafeteria. He found two skunks eating cookies (evidentaly) they had eaten alot and looked full. He called animal control right away. The workers took the skunks and (realeased) them into the woods. The smell stayed in the building for a week, until it smelled normal again.

WRITTEN EXPRESSION CONTENT UNITS SCORING FORM
Story C: "When the School Closed" (p. 73)

1. Our <u>school</u> was <u>closed</u>.	0	(1)	17. There were <u>two</u>.	0	(1)
2. It was last <u>Wednesday</u>.	0	(1)	18. They were eating <u>cookies</u>.	0	(1)
3. It was a <u>school day</u>.	(0)	1	19. They had <u>eaten many</u>.	0	(1)
4. It was <u>closed all day</u>.	0	(1)	20. They looked <u>full</u>.	0	(1)
5. The <u>janitor came in</u> at <u>6</u> <u>a.m.</u>	0	(1)	21. He called <u>animal control</u>.	0	(1)
6. He <u>opened</u> the <u>school</u>.	(0)	1	22. He called <u>right away</u>.	0	(1)
7. He <u>smelled</u> something.	0	(1)	23. The <u>workers</u> came.	0	(1)
8. It was <u>strong</u>.	0	(1)	24. They <u>took</u> the <u>skunks</u>.	0	(1)
9. It almost <u>knocked him over</u>. (figurative meaning)	0	(1)	25. They <u>let</u> them <u>go</u>.	0	(1)
10. It was a <u>skunk</u>.	0	(1)	26. It was in the <u>woods</u>.	0	(1)
11. He <u>opened</u> the <u>doors</u>.	0	(1)	27. The <u>smell stayed</u>.	0	(1)
12. He <u>left them</u> open.	0	(1)	28. It was in the <u>building</u>.	0	(1)
13. He <u>searched</u>. (looked in)	0	(1)	29. The smell <u>finally left</u>.	(0)	1
14. He looked in the <u>library</u>.	0	(1)	30. It took <u>one week</u>.	0	(1)
15. He looked in the <u>cafeteria</u>.	0	(1)	31. The <u>school</u> smelled <u>normal</u>.	0	(1)
16. He <u>found</u> the <u>skunks</u>.	0	(1)		**Content Units total**	28/31

Discourse Score	_28_ Content Units / 31 possible × 100 = _90_ % Content Included
Sentence Score	_28_ Content Units / _10_ T-units* = _2.80_ Sentence Score (record 2 decimal places)
Word Score	_88_ Total Words − _3_ Error Words = _85_ Total Correct Words / _88_ Total Words × 100 = _97_ % Words Correct

11-13

EXAMPLE 7

This example was written by a boy (age 15;11) with normal language.

> There was a building that was old, but no one knew how old it was because there were no records of it. People talked about it because it had a history. Some people knew how old it was, however. They knew that it was used in a war long ago as a hospital for (hundred) of soldiers. They were treated there but some died and were buried in the graveyard behind the building. People didn't think about the hidden graveyard and they didn't care about it. Then the city wanted land to build a new road which meant the building would be destroyed. This made people suddenly care about the building. To prevent it from being demolished, people wrote articles, gave speeches, and raised money. Eventually they saved the building and graveyard, and they also saved their history which was more important.

WRITTEN EXPRESSION CONTENT UNITS SCORING FORM
Story D: "The Building" (p. 75)

Item	0	1	Item	0	1
1. There was a building.	0	(1)	18. People did not think about it.	0	(1)
2. It was old.	0	(1)	19. It was almost hidden.	0	(1)
3. No one knew how old.	0	(1)	20. They did not care.	0	(1)
4. There were no records.	0	(1)	21. Then something happened.	(0)	1
5. People talked about it.	0	(1)	22. The city wanted the land.	0	(1)
6. It had a history.	0	(1)	23. They needed a new road.	0	(1)
7. Some people knew.	0	(1)	24. The building would be demolished.	0	(1)
8. It was used in a war.	0	(1)	25. People suddenly cared.	0	(1)
9. It was long ago.	0	(1)	26. They wrote articles.	0	(1)
10. The building was a hospital.	0	(1)	27. They gave speeches.	0	(1)
11. Soldiers came there.	0	(1)	28. They raised money.	0	(1)
12. There were hundreds.	0	(1)	29. They saved the building.	0	(1)
13. Many were treated.	0	(1)	30. They saved the graveyard.*	0	(1)
14. Many died.	0	(1)	31. They saved something else.	(0)	1
15. They were buried.	0	(1)	32. It was their history.	0	(1)
16. The graveyard was still there.*	0	(1)	33. That was more important.	0	(1)
17. It was behind the building.	0	(1)	**Content Units total**	31	/33

*Note: Count graveyard as one word when counting total words for Written Expression regardless of spacing.

Discourse Score	31 Content Units / 33 possible × 100 = 94 % Content Included
Sentence Score	31 Content Units / 14 T-units* = 2.21 Sentence Score (record 2 decimal places)
Word Score	142 Total Words − 1 Error Words = 141 Total Correct Words / 142 Total Words × 100 = 99 % Words Correct

EXAMPLE 8

This example was written by a girl (14;0) with language learning disability. The first two T-units are tricky because the student's attempt to combine them by inserting "that" is not grammatical. The examiner marked them as separate T-units to avoid overcrediting syntactic ability and circled "that" as an extraneous error word.

WRITTEN EXPRESSION CONTENT UNITS SCORING FORM
Story D: "The Building" (p. 75)

1. There was a building.	0	①	18. People did not think about it.	⓪		1
2. It was old.	⓪	1	19. It was almost hidden.	0		1
3. No one knew how old.	0	①	20. They did not care.	0		1
4. There were no records.	⓪	1	21. Then something happened.	0		1
5. People talked about it.	0	①	22. The city wanted the land.	0		1
6. It had a history.	0	①	23. They needed a new road.	0		1
7. Some people knew.	0	①	24. The building would be demolished.	0	①	
8. It was used in a war.	0	①	25. People suddenly cared.	0	①	
9. It was long ago.	⓪	1	26. They wrote articles.	0	①	
10. The building was a hospital.	⓪	1	27. They gave speeches.	0	①	
11. Soldiers came there.	0	①	28. They raised money.	0	①	
12. There were hundreds.	0	①	29. They saved the building.	0	①	
13. Many were treated.	⓪	1	30. They saved the graveyard.*	0	①	
14. Many died.	⓪	1	31. They saved something else.	⓪		1
15. They were buried.	0	①	32. It was their history.	0	①	
16. The graveyard was still there.*	0	①	33. That was more important.	⓪		1
17. It was behind the building.	0	①	**Content Units total**		19	/33

*Note: Count graveyard as one word when counting total words for Written Expression regardless of spacing.

Discourse Score	_19_ Content Units / 33 possible × 100 = _58_ % Content Included
Sentence Score	_19_ Content Units / _8_ T-units* = _2.38_ Sentence Score (record 2 decimal places)
Word Score	_72_ Total Words – _3_ Error Words = _69_ Total Correct Words / _72_ Total Words × 100 = _96_ % Words Correct